CHASING LIFE

THE REMARKABLE TRUE STORY OF LOVE, JOY, AND ACHIEVEMENT AGAINST ALL ODDS

ROBERT PARDI
and PHYLLIS MELHADO

Prominence Publishing

www.prominencepublishing.com

Chasing Life/ Robert Pardi and Phyllis Melhado. – 1st ed.

ISBN: 978-1-988925-78-3

CHASING LIFE

Praise for Chasing Life

"Cancer and death have a unique way of getting our attention. As a hospice physician, many of my patients used to tell me they became 'alive' only after facing cancer and death ... and some regretted all of the years and decades they spent 'sleep-walking.' Desiree and Rob in this book share what it means to be live fully aware, awake, and alive. If you want to live an abundant life - one that is fully woke - this book will grab, surprise, inspire, break, and renew you because everything you heard before is probably wrong. The abundant life is not about fame, money, and personal success."

James A. Avery, MD, Visiting Assistant Professor of Medicine, University of Virginia

"Love, we learn is not always about a fairy tale with happy endings. It's a tale of two people who in sharing their deepest vulnerabilities, discover each other and themselves wholeheartedly. In this vivid retelling of his 11 years caring for his wife, Robert challenges the reader to ask themselves essential life questions about how adversity calls on us to rise-up and embrace our fuller humanity. This is a story of love in its most transformative expression."

Mark Stolow, CEO, Huddol Journeys

"*Chasing Life* tells the story of two extraordinary people who, together, faced one of life's greatest challenges with grace. Robert Pardi shares his journey with his wife Dr. Desiree Pardi during which he was her warrior while she battled cancer. The lessons that Desiree learned from being both cancer patient and palliative care physician, and the many examples of Robert's path to resilience, are invaluable and should be shared with everyone. As if that isn't enough, this story is about much more; it is about great love. Robert and Desiree lived that love to the end, and by doing so set not only the example but also the bar for all us."

Trish Humenansky-Laub, Founder of Comfort in Their Journey LLC and Author of the *Comfort in Their Journey* Book Series

"Chasing Life is a heartbreaking and heartwarming story about two amazing individuals, Desiree and Rob, who shared the passion for life through transformative love and angelic compassion in the face of horrendous circumstances. Undaunted in her dedication to care for the suffering, while going through 11 years of her own recurring and worsening cancer, Desiree gave the full energy of her heart and soul to helping people with advanced illness. As a physician, she was an early champion of palliative care, and was able to help so many people through the most difficult times of their lives. All the while, Rob's inspirational, relentless support and devotion were a testament to the meaning of genuine love."

Csaba Mera, MD - built the nation's first healthplan-based palliative care program.

"Chasing Life is a love story, an ode to a brilliant doctor whose own illness shaped a legacy of patient care that I have surely benefited from in my own cancer journey. This memoir proves that luck goes beyond issues of mortality - that the greater gift is to be lucky in love."

Leslie Lehr, Author of *A Boob's Life: How America's Obsession Shaped Me...and You*....and breast cancer survivor.

"*Chasing Life* is a the beautifully written story of a vibrant young couple rising in their careers and enjoying life, until a diagnosis of terminal cancer invades their lives. The journey of Desiree and Robert Pardi will inspire and guide couples facing cancer and other serious disease and teach them how to approach each day with hope, determination and purpose. Patients facing end of life will also be inspired to learn how Dr. Desiree Pardi persevered through medical school and her residency living with stage four metastatic breast cancer, and then chose to give back with the time she had left as a palliative care physician, especially as Director of Palliative Medicine at Weill-Cornell Hospital.

Chasing Life is a true love story about two people committed to each other that should be read by everyone and its messages embraced."

Bob Kieserman, Executive Director, The Power of the Patient Project: The National Library of Patient Rights and Advocacy

"Inner strength, the drive to embrace life regardless of circumstances, a heart of gold. Both Desiree and Rob seemed to share these values, forever binding them at a depth that knew no limits. The courage to dig deep into the conflicts that define all of our lives is a courage that is rarely known. Desiree and Rob discovered these conflicts, as well as the emotional obstacle course they create in our path. How many of us, when faced with life's most jagged obstacles, can maintain our values while learning our final lessons? This book is both a reminder and an inspiration as we struggle to move through our own major barricades."

Patty Civalleri, Author, *Becoming Trader Joe*

"Chasing life - when you know what you love, you know who you are. A vivid manifesto of the healing power of connecting to life through love. The kind of love that enriches the soul. A reflection on resilience, impermanence and the preciousness of the here and now."

Dana Tarcatu, MD, VNSNY Hospice and Palliative Care, New York, NY

"This beautiful memoir is a testament of what it takes to have true love and selfless partnership through adversity, heart break and triumph. Most importantly, it demonstrates how we can make a huge impact in another person's life and how embracing all that life gives us shows us our true purpose even beyond '*love at last sight*'."

Brenda Blais Nesbitt, Coaching for Caregivers Canada

"Told with luminous and heartbreaking prose, *Chasing Life* is a story about hope, courage, and thankfulness in the face of a terminal cancer diagnosis. Desiree's incredible grace and her husband Robert's staunch loyalty are both an inspiration and a testament to true love."

Anita Hughes, Author of *A Magical New York Christmas*

"Truly a love story for the 21st century, *Chasing Life* portrays the life and death of Dr. Des Pardi and the unflinching love of her husband Rob. While *Chasing Life* is a love story on par with *Love Story*, the book and the movie from 1970, it adds another dimension to love, one that involves more than just the couple at the heart of the story. This book should be read by anyone in love, aspiring to be in love, or looking to a future in compassionate health care."

Elizabeth Coplan, Founder and Chief Playwright, Grief Dialogues Health Care Education

"*Chasing Life* is an incredibly powerful story. Desiree and Rob are each energetic, brilliant individuals, committed to each other and to life, joining forces to face Desiree's agonizing illness. Truly a story of love, persistence and resilience."

Regina McBride, author of *Ghost Songs* and *The Nature of Water and Air*

"This is a love story and like so many caregiving journeys, is guided by the desire to make the life of someone who is struggling with an illness as full as it can possibly be. As a cancer survivor myself, I marvel at the strength and determination Desiree possessed, while clearly understanding her time here was short. This is not only a story for caregivers and patients, this is a story for anyone who believes or wants to believe, extraordinary people and great love and devotion exist. Robert Pardi has written a beautiful tribute to his incredible wife and shared it with the world as a message of love and hope."

Michelle Chaffee, Founder & CEO alska

"Living with stage four metastatic breast cancer, Director of Palliative Medicine at Weill-Cornell Hospital, Dr. Desiree Pardi knew what her end would look like. Her unique approach to managing adversity inspired countless patients and friends. She chose compassion and love over fear and anger. Let the wisdom and love in this book transform you."

Catherine Gaynor, MA, Theology

"It seems like an oxymoron to say that *Chasing Life* is both tragic and uplifting, but this riveting tale of love and devotion through heartbreaking times is a blueprint for how we should all live our lives."

Charles Salzberg, twice Shamus Award nominated and Beverly Hills Book Award winner for *Second Story Man* and *Swann's Last Song.*

"Robert Pardi and Phyllis Melhado have written Robert's moving and beautiful true love story that is riveting, inspiring, emotional, and embracing. Despite tragedy and heartbreak, they show that love can prevail in the best and darkest of times through determination and resiliency. A must read for all who love, want to be loved, and are loved."

MaryAnn Ragone DeLambily, MAS, MPH President,
MRD Consulting, LLC

"*Chasing Life* is a powerful and poignant true story about love, life, death, and choice. Using an unconventional approach to managing her cancer diagnosis, Dr. Des Pardi teaches us the importance of respecting the patient's values at life's end, even when they differ from our own. In this fast and captivating read, Chasing Life will inspire you to appreciate the smaller gifts in life, encourage you to contemplate your own mortality, and challenge you to fully embrace the importance of patient autonomy at life's end."

Kim Callinan, President & CEO of Compassion & Choices

The purpose of life is to live it, to taste experience to the utmost, to reach out eagerly and without fear for newer and richer experience

Eleanor Roosevelt

In Loving Memory of
Desiree Ann Pardi

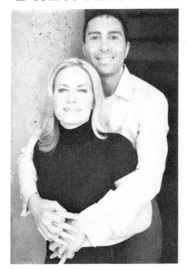

Foreword

Chasing Life... I have been thinking a lot about the word "chasing." It is one of my toddler granddaughter's favorite words as she runs around acting like she hopes that someone will catch up to her but truly wishing she will outsmart whoever is behind her and stay in the lead.

You are about to read a love story, a story of triumph, a story of drive, passion, compassion and about a courageous fight in the face of adversity. I came to know Dr. Desiree Pardi as someone who was always chasing her dream; she did not just pursue the dream in order to catch up; she caught up with her dream, outsmarted that dream and pursued another, and another, and another. Chasing Life is the perfect title for this labor of love, a portrait of an incredible young woman pursuing her passion, surpassing every expectation and then moving forward again until she could go no further because of a devastating and aggressive disease. But anyone who met Desiree casually would never have known any of that. Her cheerful countenance, her enthusiasm, her bright smile never betrayed the battle she was fighting or her drive to satisfy her curiosity, create new scientific knowledge or take exceptional care of her patients.

I met Desiree when she was a medical student, and although I was aware of who she was during the PhD phase of her training, I got to know her and her spirited and devoted husband, Robert, as she planned her return to clinical training after her PhD was completed. She confided to me that she had a medical problem, disclosed her diagnosis, and questioned whether she could and should continue her studies. I saw her drive and her need for normalcy, but much more than that, I saw someone who knew that she, herself, could make a difference and she was motivated to continue her studies at whatever cost. And make no mistake: the training is tough. Sometimes it is an eighty-hour work-week, and some days can be fifteen hours on your feet in the Operating Room. But Desiree was determined - with the condition that no one be apprised of her condition. She wanted no special treatment and most especially, no pity. My role would be to make sure she was able to go to her medical appointments as necessary by approving schedule modifications. To me that was routine—and those types of accommodations continue to be common to support students' wellness.

Throughout my career, I remember hearing the mantra: "the patient has the problem." I was taught as a clinician, to care deeply about my patients but in some way to create boundaries to be able to live my own life. It is inevitable that certain patients "follow" you home in your mind and in your thoughts. So is it also true that those of us who care about students often "bring our students home with us" and we are touched by their circumstances and try to imagine the optimal way to be of help. Desiree touched my spirit in this way. I did not do anything special for her; in fact, she did something special for me. She inspired me to overlook minor irritations and focus on the big picture. She inspired me to be grateful. I wish I could have done more to help her but was reassured of her outstanding clinical care and I could see first-hand that she was well cared for by Robert, so much so that I began to worry about him!

I was surprised to learn that just prior to medical school graduation, Desiree was in a small group and she stunned her classmates (many of whom did not know her well since she was out of sync due to her PhD training) by recounting her story. It was a powerful disclosure and something her classmates would never forget. Graduation day was memorable for me. As Desiree walked across the stage and I had the honor to place the MD hood over her head, my eyes filled with tears of pride and joy, knowing the depth of the moment and with hope for the future.

I followed Desiree's career journey from afar and we stayed in touch. I had heard about the impactful and transformational talk she was preparing for the VNA (which you will read about in Chapter 31), and I asked her if she would be willing to be the speaker for our White Coat Ceremony (a rite of passage for first year medical students) for the incoming Class of 2009. She was super excited about this opportunity to greet new matriculants as they traversed the stage to be "coated" with their first White Coat, and for the very first time, commit to and say the "Oath." Desiree informed me that she was open to discussing her personal journey and she would think about what she wanted to share with future doctors emphasizing empathy, listening and patient autonomy. Several weeks before the event I reached out to Desiree and upon getting no response I became concerned. Robert subsequently contacted me to inform me that Desiree was admitted to the hospital and that things were not looking good... Desiree never gave that speech. One of her colleagues had the challenging role of speaking in her stead after we announced that Desiree had passed away that very week. I sat next to Robert in the audience during that ceremony and all I could think about was the loss of such an amazing person: brilliant, selfless, compassionate, generous, thoughtful, caring, and loving.

Desiree surrounds me every day, not just in the assortment of turtles she gifted me for my collection – which bring smiles - but more importantly, by gifting me a sense of purpose, inspiration and drive. There is a Talmudic quote that goes as follows:

I have learned much from my teachers and even more from my friends, but from my students I have learned more than from all of them.

Rabbi Hanina, Babylonian Talmud, Tractate Ta'anit 7a

Desiree, who was my student, became my teacher. Her lessons will continue to live on as I pass on the lessons I have learned to other students and mentees. It is a perpetual gift as these lessons will be passed forward. This is a monumental influence with immeasurable impact. It is my hope that through your reading this inspirational story of love, hope, dreams, and courage that you will learn from Desiree and from Robert and that you, too, will help to perpetuate these important lessons, lessons of caring for others, listening, enjoying the moment, and appreciation, among many others.

With gratitude to Desiree and to Robert for their gifts of friendship, learning and love,

Suzi Rose

Pacentro, Italy - 2021

I never believed in love at first sight. It's a total illusion. But ask me about love at last sight. That's a whole other story.

New York - 2009

I am in Mount Sinai hospital, sitting at the foot of my wife's bed. She looks so sweet and beautiful. Desiree was a beauty, plain and simple - beauty then, and beauty now, even though she has fallen into what is medically called a uremia induced sleep.

I've learned a lot about dying patients over the last few years and I know it won't be long now. I already carried out her wishes. I know the path I have paved. I know this from the countless number of times my award-winning, palliative care physician wife tended to dying patients. Now another palliative care physician is tending to her.

But what I know most of all is that I love this woman in gut-wrenching, non-quantifiable ways and have for twenty-four years, including nearly twenty years of marriage, a marriage which covered extraordinary terrain, was filled with joy even in the darkest of times and melded our two lives together in ways far removed from anything either of us could ever have imagined on that day we met in 1985.

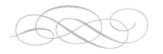

Chapter 1

B ack in '85, Stony Brook University was a great place to go to school - nice campus, excellent teachers, and a great mix of students. It was pure nirvana for an Italian kid from Long Island, like me.

It was late August, students were returning, and there was some serious partying going on. All my friends were checking out the new crop of freshman girls, but I wasn't too interested because I had my eye on a girl that I'd met the semester before. Lisa was a real Wasp princess from Connecticut, the kind whose daddy would probably not be too happy having me in the picture, but I was pretty sure she liked me and I had high hopes for connecting later that night at the party where everyone was going.

Heading back to the dorm, I ran into a buddy who was fixated on some redhead sunning herself on a nearby slope. Brian was taking drags on his cigarette, salivating through his clouds of smoke.

"Yo - numb nuts, get rid of that thing in your mouth," I called out. "It'll kill you." Back then, smoking was still too cool to be recognized as the killer that we now know it is, but I was pre-med, and in that group, none of us smoked. We had read the studies and we knew. I was talking to a wall, however. Brian was riveted.

"I'm busy," he mumbled, as he dragged on his cigarette, never taking his eyes off the girl on the slope.

I glanced over at her and laughed. She was a real looker, and there was no way she was going to hook up with Brian, who was on the chubby side and had yet to conquer his teenage acne.

"Give it a rest," I told him. "She's definitely outta your league."

"Hey, a guy can dream, can't he?"

Dream on, I thought, laughing. "Will I see you at Vic's tonight?"

"Will there be women and booze?"

"Is the Pope Catholic?"

I was still laughing as I made my way to my dorm. I could party with the best of them and I was really looking forward to the evening. The hallway was crowded with students, including a couple of hot-looking chicks making their way to the rooms that would be their homes for the next several months. When I reached mine and opened the door, I was pretty pleased with myself. It wasn't the train wreck that some of my friends' rooms were. My desk was organized with my Smith Corona portable in the center, textbooks piled neatly on one side and my cassette player on the other. The tapes weren't in any particular order, but I knew how to find the Madonna – on whom I had a serious crush, back then - Led Zeppelin, and Bon Jovi in a pinch.

I had practically worn the Madonna tape out, so I thought I would listen to Bon Jovi. As I walked over to my desk, I sensed something in the room. I swung around. My radar was right. There *was* something in my room - or rather, someone. It was a girl, and she was lying on my bed. And holy shit - was she ever hot: hippee-looking, with long blonde hair, an innocent face, and a killer body in tight, short shorts. She was wearing a tie-dyed halter top that kind of reverberated as she breathed in and out, showcasing her God-given abundance. Who needed weed? I could have stared at that for hours.

"And then she spoke.

"Hey...how's your day going?" she asked as if we were old friends.

How's my day going? "Excuse me," I managed to get out. I wasn't as quick on the uptake as I usually was. I was too busy focusing on that halter top and what it was covering. "Uh, what are you doing here?" I asked with as straight a face as I could muster.

"Well, I'm here because I saw you out there before," she said pointing to the window, "and I thought you were cute, so I followed you."

Followed me? I had to admit to myself that I was flattered. She was a great-looking girl - a little ballsy, perhaps, but great looking.

"So what's your name?" I asked.

"Desiree. Desiree Ann Flannery," she said with the sweetest possible voice. That voice in no way matched the body, and I really didn't know what to make of her. She was disarming.

She popped up and gave me one hell of a seductive smile. "So tell me about you," she said.

"Well, I have a feeling you already know who I am. You found my room, didn't you?"

She laughed, throwing her head back confidently. "OK, busted, Mr. Robert Pardi, Jr., who, by the way, looks pretty grown up to be a junior." Then she looked me up and down, very, very slowly.

I was hard pressed to speak.

"Well, anyway," she went on, "I figured that since I'm freshman pre-med, it might help to get to know a sophomore pre-med." She paused. "I thought it could really be fun going over labs with you." She followed that with another one of those smiles.

Labs, uh... "Look, Desiree, I'd love to chat, but I'm going out soon and I've really gotta get ready."

She leaned back flirtatiously.

Well, she was really a knockout, but I had set my goal the semester before and had spent the whole summer thinking about Lisa and how I was finally going to reel her in and, at that point, I really needed to get ready.

"Look, I'm in a rush. Gotta jump into the shower."

She made no move to leave.

"I really need to get undressed now..."

"Feel free," she said, lounging back on the bed.

It was clear she was not about to leave, so I took off my shirt, jeans and Jockeys, and quickly wrapped a towel around myself. She watched every motion but didn't say a word.

"Take it easy," I said, and headed for the men's shower room. *Who was this girl?* I laughed to myself as I walked down the hall.

The shower room was empty. I picked the stall on the end, turned the water on full force and hopped in. It felt good. So did thoughts of Lisa. Yes sir. This was going to be *the* night.

"So what do I need to know about my first semester?"

What?

I pulled the curtain open and there she was, Desiree Ann Flannery, sitting on the bench opposite, talking as if we were still in my room and I still had on all my clothes.

"I mean, do I really have to tough it out and study all the time, or is there time to have some...you know...fun?"

Was this girl serious? "Uh, you DO know I'm naked in this shower."

"Well, I pretty much saw everything before..." she laughed.

Hmm, I thought, smiling to myself. *Guess she liked what she saw...*

"Look. I need you to do two things right now. First, hand me a towel. And second, get the hell out! If they catch you in here, I could lose my housing."

We looked at each other for a long second, then she threw me a towel.

"Well," she said, shrugging her shoulders, "guess I'll just see you later at the party."

She got up and opened the door to leave. Then she turned around, shot me a dazzling smile and in a flash left me standing there, dripping, and shaking my head.

What was the story with this girl? Maybe I should ditch Lisa and call her back, she really is smokin hot.

I took a few deep breaths, slaved over my long, curly black hair, poured myself into tight jeans and my best t-shirt and left for the evening I'd been thinking about for weeks.

The party was in a senior's apartment off campus, and by the time I got there, it was wall-to-wall kids downing beer and vodka mixes and smoking grass. Springsteen's "Born in the US" was blasting. I made my way through the crowd and spotted Lisa standing around with two other girls.

She shot me a smile. I shot her one back.

Yes! I thought. *I'm in!*

The music segued into Frankie Goes to Hollywood's "Relax," that year's primer on how to get it on. The dance floor was crowded with gyrating couples. I zeroed in on Lisa and pulled her onto the dance floor. I pushed closer to her and was feeling pretty damned good. It was all going as planned.

Suddenly I felt someone grab me from behind and start pushing into my body. Without looking, I was quite sure I knew who it was. I turned around and yup. It was my shower buddy, and she was raring to go in tight jeans and a sweater cut down to there. But it was her eyes. There was no mistaking how she was looking at me and it was beyond a turn-on. Never in my wildest dreams did I ever think I would ever have had a choice to make between two fabulous women, both so different but both so hot - but that move of Desiree's really got to me and I found myself whispering "sorry" in Lisa's ear and turning to give Desiree Ann Flannery my full attention.

"See you around," I heard Lisa say matter-of-factly, but I barely noticed. I was already charting a new course with the smokin' Irish girl who clearly wanted to be with me. And if the way she danced was any indication, I was in for the time of my life.

Everyone pulled back to watch as we went at it, and about a half hour of that was about all we could handle and it wasn't long until we raced back to my dorm. Well, "racing" is putting a generous spin on it. We'd both had a lot to drink - Blue Whales, as I recall, a lethal combination of vodka, liqueur and fruit juices that make you think you were just having a morning eye-opener.

We stumbled back to the dorm, falling all over each other, laughing till it hurt. When we finally got to my door, we fell into the room and then onto the floor. I can't remember ever having laughed so much in my life...the weed and the booze and this girl who, against my will, had totally turned my head around.

After rolling around on the floor, I got up and helped her to the bed. Nicholas Cage, by the way, totally stole "I'm taking you to the bed," from me when he used it on Cher in Moonstruck two years later.

Nick notwithstanding, I managed to get us both on the bed. I remember nosing into her neck and groping around some...and then...*nada*. I passed out. Cold. After all of that, my big night ended with a total bust - no pun intended. Out there on the dance floor I was so sure the night was going to end with a nice notch on my belt, but the only thing I had to show for my efforts the next morning was a big, ugly, red hickey.

But this girl really liked me and over the next couple of weeks, we spent lots of time together, mostly talking and just having fun. As it turned out, I didn't actually "score" for several days. Desiree may have had the face of an angel and a killer body, but it proved to be her mind that made me want to be with her. She was so damned smart and so interested in just about everything. I had never met a girl, or a guy, for that matter, who had such broad-based intellectual curiosity. There didn't seem to be a topic about which she didn't want to know more - cultures in different parts of the world, the history of the U.S., fishing villages, how bathrooms on boats worked, animals of every kind, what it was like to grow old.

She was observant, insightful, hungry for information about everyone and everything. In high school, she studied Latin because she wanted to understand the roots of so many languages. And then she studied Judaism, because she went to school with so many Jewish kids and wanted to know more about them.

And she challenged me at every turn, which, as an Italian-American, was the total opposite of most of the women I had been surrounded by growing up. I was a fan of Reagan's, for example, and when I said I thought he was terrific, she roared.

"Ronald Reagan? He's a joke! His economics are just for the rich, and there are too many disenfranchised people out there."

Well, coming from a strictly Republican family, it had never occurred to me to look at him from another perspective. And when I told her that I didn't really like chemistry, was having misgivings about medical school, and was going just because my family thought it would be great to be able to boast about me becoming a doctor, she was indignant.

"Don't do something just because somebody else wants you to do it. You have the right to choose - and don't ever forget it! It's your life. Do something that you really want to do." She paused. "I would never give up my right to choose. Ever."

"Yeah," I admitted. "Med school's not my choice. What I really want is just to make money."

"Money? Ugh," she grunted. "You may be cute, but that's a really selfish way to think. There's more to life than money. You could do something noble. Think about all the people in the world who are not as lucky as we are." She paused. "I'm seriously thinking about going to work for Doctors Without Borders after I finish my medical studies."

Doctors Without Borders? Gee-sus. Mother Theresa with a killer body! Her predilection for low pay and terrible working conditions notwithstanding, the fact that she had such strong opinions about everything was a real turn on. She even had a different take on the music we both liked.

"Pink Floyd is more than just music to get high to, Robert! Did you ever really stop to listen to the words?"

Frankly, up until then, I hadn't, but Desiree pointed out that Pink Floyd was talking about society and things that were not right. Coming from a home where my parents rarely discussed anything and where it was thought that women's opinions were not especially relevant, it was a whole new world for me. She opened up my thinking in so many ways, and it had a powerful effect. She admitted that even though it went against her beliefs that you should do only what you really want to do, she had actually gotten engaged to a guy she had been dating because her need to get her parents to love her had clouded her decision-making process. Her parents had married very young - both of them were 18 - and Desiree felt they had the same expectations of her.

"I was kind of hoping that over time it would just dissipate, and that Tommy and I would go our separate ways, but the minute I saw you...well, knew I had to make that break right away," she said.

I was totally up ended. The poor guy had actually given her a ring - but she gave it back and told him it was over. I felt bad for him, but his loss sure as hell was my gain, and after a couple of weeks of what we used to call "messing around," one night in the bottom of her bunk bed when her roommates were out, we gave ourselves to each other and it was worth every minute of all the teasing and waiting. Desiree Ann Flannery was the whole package, and I was hooked.

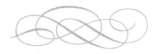

Chapter 2

They always say that things happen when you least expect it. Well, the last thing I expected was to meet someone like Desiree and I sure as hell didn't expect to fall in love. I didn't even want to. I was 19 years old and really hadn't had all that much experience, despite my tough-talking, fast-on-the-uptake, bad-boy mouth. Moreover, my parents' marriage hadn't set a great example for me, and I had pretty much vowed I would be a desert island.

Despite my air of self-confidence, underneath it all I was still severely wounded from a difficult relationship I had had with my abusive, gambling addicted, alcoholic father. Aside from physical beatings while I was growing up, he did his best to stifle any semblance of self-esteem I tried to develop. I had had to work really hard to develop that self-esteem and become resilient, and actually had come to even be thankful for the lessons I learned that would enable me to confront things thrown at me. By the time I got to college, I was so much better than I had been - but still working on it - and I couldn't believe that after learning who I really was, Des still picked me, well more like stalked me - but I thank God every day of my life that she did. This beyond smart, funny, gorgeous girl who could have had anybody - absolutely anybody - miraculously wanted me and my body, and as much as I thought I would never want a committed relationship, a little voice in the back of my mind kept nagging at me: *Boy - if you even think about letting this woman go, you are out of your friggin' mind. This one has your number and let's just let her keep it.*

The way she expanded my world and made me think differently about things made a profound change in my life. Des was the antithesis of the women in my traditional Italian-American family. When she felt it was appropriate, she spoke her mind and made me think beyond the somewhat constricted view I had not realized I had about many things. And it was exciting! Getting to know her confirmed my decision about switching out of pre-med. Des was the stuff doctors should be made of. Not me. I felt I was far better suited to chasing the almighty dollar and viewed it as a way of distancing myself from my father. Acknowledging that and moving on was a huge relief. Des gave me the confidence to follow my own path...to be "me."

And the fun we had together! We laughed, we played. I was so alive when I was with her. Who wouldn't want all that? ˙

About six weeks in, I decided to tell my mother that I'd met the girl. I remember calling her from a pay phone in my dorm hall. Des was excited, hanging on my back and snuggling in.

The conversation started off fine.

"Yes, Mom. Everything's good - actually really good."

I could tell by her long, contented sigh that my mother liked that.

"Listen," I went on, "uh, there's a girl I'd like to bring home to meet you."

That didn't go over quite so well. There was a long silence, then she asked what the girl's name was.

"Desiree."

Another silence, and then my mom started fishing. She couldn't come right out and ask me if her deepest, darkest fears about her baby boy falling prey to the lures of a non-Italian or, heaven-forbid, someone whose skin was a shade darker than Mediterranean olive, had come to pass.

"So," she asked, "what color are her eyes?"

"What color are her eyes? Mom! What difference does that make?"

"What color?"

"They're blue, Mom."

I could sense some relief on the other end, although I knew she was hoping for the miracle of Frank Sinatra blue eyes that came with a name like Rinaldi, DeMarco or Carbone.

"She's Irish, Mom, and I'd like for you and Dad and Nonna Mary to meet her." My grandmother had protected me my whole life. I knew she wouldn't fail me now - even though in her day, marrying out of the clan was a sure way to be not-so-subtly reviled by all of your relatives for the rest of your life.

I could practically hear the *agita* gurgling up from my mother's stomach.

She cleared her throat, then ventured: "Is it serious?"

I jumped right back in there. "Yes, Mom. It's serious."

At this point, I could hear my father in the background, wanting to know what was going on. My father and I were in a permanent state of civil war, which only got worse as the years went by. Nothing I did was right enough for him and hooking up with Des would certainly fall into that category. We may have been at huge odds, but at that point in time, despite the fact I did not like or respect him, I still had this need to show him that I was worthy...that there was somebody out there who really loved me, and especially someone as amazing as Des. Having my parents meet her took on outsize proportions.

"And then my mother said exactly what I expected her to say: "But Robert, there are so many nice Italian girls out there."

Yeah, yeah, yeah...

"I know there are lots of nice Italian girls out there, Mom, but I'm grown up now, and this is the girl for me."

Then I got *The Sigh*. Yes - that one - that unique form of breath control mothers use when they are feeling extra noble because they're letting their kid do something that they really don't want them to do.

But on that day, my mother did the right thing - or so I thought - by suggesting that I bring Des over to the house for Sunday dinner.

"She invited me to dinner?" Des's face gleamed with a wonderful little girl type look she had when she was especially happy.

She squeezed my hand, then reached up and kissed me on the cheek. The smile, however, was short lived.

"Guess now we've gotta tackle the Irish contingent."

So we switched places - Des on the phone, me holding on from the back, arms around her waist. By then she had told me that she often felt at odds with her mother. I knew how difficult that could be because of my own relationship with my father.

"Great. Everything's great, Mom...Yes, I'm doing really well with my classes."

Des pushed against me for support.

"Listen...I met a guy." Pause. "Oh, a few weeks ago."

She ground into me which felt peculiarly calming considering that the same thing in other circumstances made me as raring to go as a stallion in a brood mare's paddock.

"No, Mom. That's over. Tommy and I broke up."

A really long pause, this time.

"It doesn't matter, Mom. He really wasn't the right one - now I know that for sure....yes...yes...Robert. His name is Robert Pardi, Junior."

Pause.

"Italian. It's an Italian name."

I thought I could hear her mother groan.

Des moved the phone away from her ear and turned to look at me. She loved her mother and didn't want to disappoint her. But she loved me as well.

"Yeah, I know, Mom."

Des had warned me that the call might be a little tough because one of their relatives had married an Italian and he'd had an affair, leaving the women in the family a bit circumspect when it came to Italian men.

"Well, Mom, I promise you. This Italian is quite wonderful!"

There was a pause and I could hear her mother clearing her throat, but couldn't make out what she said next.

"Yes, I really want you to meet Robert. I'd like to bring him over one Sunday."

We breathed sighs of relief: both families were now duly apprized. We were on our way to being officially "serious."

The following Sunday afternoon, we got into my old Valero and drove out to Hicksville to do battle on the 100 per cent Italian front.

For starters, you need to know that the Sunday meal is a big deal in an Italian family, with grandparents, aunts and uncles and a bunch of kids around the table. It's usually served around three in the afternoon and is pretty much a feast which almost always includes some kind of meat dish and pasta with gravy which most people call "sauce" but Italians - especially those whose ancestors come from southern Italy or Sicily - call "gravy."

We pulled up to the house and went up to the front door. I held Des's hand and could feel her anxiety.

"Not to worry, Baby. They'll love you!" I said as I squeezed her fingers with one hand and rang the bell with the other.

My mother must have been standing right there because the door opened in a nano-second. She smiled. "And in case Des didn't already know we were Italian, we could hear Sinatra crooning "My Way" on the stereo.

My mother leaned over and planted a kiss on my cheek, then pulled back and looked at Des, an excruciatingly long look from Des's sandals up her tight-fitting jeans to her totally filled out halter top and the feathered earrings that peeked out from under her luscious, long, blonde hair. Yup. No Italian *ragazza*, this one.

"So this must be Desiree. Nice to meet you, dear." She gave Des her best smile.

The Sunday supper odors came wafting out. It was a smell that bore absolutely no resemblance to the meatballs and spaghetti I had told Des to expect.

I glanced at Des. She was giving my Mom her biggest smile back.

"It's so nice to meet you, Mrs. Pardi. I have really been looking forward to coming here today. Your supper smells delicious!"

"Yes," my mother said. "I've made something special, in your honor."

My parents' house was typical Long Island Italian - lots of mass-produced "art" on the walls, lamps with too many hanging crystals and ornate, curly-cue furniture with plastic covers on the cushions. The dining room table was set with big bowls of salad, plates of hard cheese, prosciutto and olives and a decanter of red wine.

Even though we weren't close back then, I was expecting to see my brother Michael, but he wasn't there because, I later learned, they hadn't told him. Hmm. So there was just my father, already at the table, drinking his martini. God forbid he should wait for everyone.

I made the introduction.

"So, you must be Dez-zer-ay," my old man said, slurring his words. Gee-sus. How many had he already had? "No, Pops," I was tempted to say. "She's Sister Mary Margaret from St. Benedict's. Decided to take the day off and come with me for a walk on the wild side."

He looked Des over but didn't say a word. He was probably sizing her up and making a mental list of things he didn't like. I could have brought Marilyn Monroe home and he would have found fault with my choice.

After an uncomfortable silence, we went into the kitchen to say hello to my Grandmother Mary, who was sitting at the table, knitting an afghan.

"Nice to meet you, Desi dear," she said with a big, warm smile. God bless Grandma Mary. I could always count on her.

Then my mother came in and went straight to the oven.

"Come have a look," she said.

Des and I walked over to her. My mother opened the oven door, and we were hit with the very strong, unmistakable odor of lamb. We looked down, and there, in a roasting pan, nestled sadly in a bed of potatoes and parsley, were four little lamb's heads, eyes wide open.

Des gagged.

"It's *Capozzelli Di Angnelli*," my mother explained. "A real Italian specialty. We made it in your honor."

It was not the thing to make for someone who had never imagined that civilized people ate such things. I could hear my father laughing from the other room.

"No way I can eat this," Des said in my ear. "No way," she repeated and squeezed my hand so hard I thought it would turn black and blue.

Even though I actually liked that lamb dish, I totally understood. It was hardly what most people would even contemplate eating - the head of an animal with the tongue, eyes and brains included. To this day I think "Mom, what the hell were you thinking?"

"Not to worry, Baby," I said, looking at my mother, who knew that I wasn't especially pleased with her at that moment. "I'll make you something you can eat."

My mother shot me a look back. Her son was going to cook for a woman. *What kind of man had she raised?*

Des gave me a big smile. She was not about to let them get to her. Nor was I.

"You know I'll always try to make things perfect for you," I said.

We both liked pasta and butter so I made us some, but I also reached over for some lamb.

My mother watched me with an undeniable smirk of satisfaction, then looked over at Des. "I knew Robert would eat the lamb. He loves my cooking. Do you know how to cook Italian, dear? Robert likes real Italian food."

There was a pause after that, but Des handled it perfectly. She just smiled, and changed the conversation, going on to tell them about her plans to for medical school.

"I've wanted to be a doctor ever since I was a little kid," she said, eyes sparkling. "My sisters' favorite toys were dolls, but mine were always my toy stethoscope and pretend doctor's bag."

"Ooh. Medical school," my father said. "You'll need loads of money for that."

He looked at me as though shooting off a warning shot: *You'll need that, too, kiddo, 'cause it's not coming from me.* I knew early on that I couldn't rely on my father for money or much of anything else, for that matter. After all his drinking and gambling, there was hardly a chance that there would be any money to help me with med school tuition. *You're in for a surprise, Pops,* I laughed to myself, as I looked back at him. I hadn't felt it necessary, at that point, to inform my family that I had just switched out of pre-med in favor of economics - and how great it felt to make a choice of my own.

"Desiree's not going to have any problems with tuition money," I chimed in.

"Oh, no," Des said quite confidently. "I'm quite sure I'll be getting scholarships and grants."

"Brains and beauty," my father said with no lack of sarcasm. It was clear that this girl was different from any girl my parents had ever imagined I might bring home, not that they imagined I would be bringing anyone home at that point, let alone a 17-year-old girl who was so resolute about her path ahead, so unlike most Italian girls, who were yet to embrace the "having it all" attitude about life. This girl was smart, was going to have a career <u>and</u> a husband - and she had gumption. I think they begrudgingly liked that, but I was only 19 and I know that they felt I was way too young to be getting seriously involved with any girl, especially one so young.

And so, we got through the meal and got my family out of the way. Next, it was my turn to meet her family. How bad could it be? A little corned beef and cabbage, maybe. I could handle that.

A couple of weeks later, we drove to a middle-class suburb where her parents lived. Their house didn't scream "Irish," but you just knew it was.

"Sure hope this starts off easier than it did at my house," I said.

Des squeezed my hand. "Not to worry. They'll love you from the moment they see you!"

I wasn't so sure.

She rang the bell and a slender woman, mid-30's, opened the door. It was her mother Dianne - and I couldn't believe how young she was! Des had told me that her parents married as teenagers, but seeing her mother was still startling.

"Hi Mom!" Des said as she hugged her. Her mother looked over Des's shoulder and focused on me.

"So," she said. "You must be Robert." She broke from Des's embrace.

We just stood there looking at one another for what seemed like an eternity. I was surprised at her youthful, flower child appearance. She looked more like she would be Des's sister, than her mother... and I think she was surprised at my whole preppie thing.

We finally smiled at each other and then Des spoke up. "Come on. Let's go in. I'm sure dinner is getting cold by now."

Whatever was in there getting cold didn't smell especially good to my Italian nose. I had been spoiled growing up with my mother and grandmother, who regularly turned out amazing, traditional Italian food. Great cooking was their calling in life. Des had told me that her mom was not especially interested in cooking. She was a nurse. That was *her* calling.

I peeked in behind Dianne and locked eyes with Des's father. He was relaxing in his Barca-lounger across the room in the corner. A large Sacred Heart of Jesus was hanging perilously close to his head.

He waved hello, and I waved back.

Des sighed then nudged me through the door.

I walked over to him and we shook hands. I grasped his hand. He grasped harder.

As we shook hands, I looked up at Jesus. *Pardon me, Lord, but I hope this doesn't turn out to be the dinner from Hell!*

I swear to you, Jesus looked back at me and winked.

Their house was pleasant, filled with light oak furniture and there were old Yankee type curtains on the windows. And the food was good - baked ham, lots of potatoes, gobs of mayo, green beans and generous servings of beer.

Both Des's mother and father were nice to me, for sure, but I suppose I was nervous and felt out of my element. I was also a bit on edge because Des had prepped me about a family dynamic that was difficult for her. She had told me that while she was sure her parents loved her very much, she always felt they paid much more attention to her sister and it made her feel bad. They may not have realized it, but she said she never felt *recognized* by them. Whenever she talked about it, there was so much sadness in her voice.

Des's sister was a year younger, and nothing like her and I did see that the attention was often redirected toward her. Looking back, perhaps it was because Des was such a star, and her parents didn't feel she needed pats on the head while they treated her sister as if she did. I didn't fully understand it, but it did seem that they were overcompensating. I did learn later about some childhood situations that could have exacerbated this tendency. And then there was the other "sibling," a friend of her sister's who had come to live with the family. She wasn't there, that first time, but on most other times when we visited, she was. Des's parents paid lots of attention to her, too, or so it seemed, but perhaps Des had predisposed me to see it that way. I can see that this was done to help the girls develop and maintain good self-esteem, yet there was unseen collateral damage for Desiree. Now, when I look back, I realize what an incredibly loving and generous thing it was to do - to take someone into their home and treat them as family. But no matter how loving the motivation was, Des had become acutely sensitive to what she saw as their perceived favoritism for the other two girls which took a toll on her. That first night I could feel it too, because whenever Des felt slighted, she squeezed my hand, under the table, and that night she squeezed my hand several times.

Des had told me that whenever she brought home all A's, which was almost always, there was no fan fair about her grades. Maybe they just expected it from her because she always excelled, but when her sister got a B, Des remarked that they couldn't say enough about how good her sister was. Nor, she said, was there really ever a "Des, dear, you look so pretty today." She always looked gorgeous, by the way! She just remembered what she perceived as criticisms. "Why are you wearing your hair that way?" and "That sweater isn't the right color for you. You should wear pastels, not that awful olive green." Her mother was into that "season" color thing that was popular back then, where some guru had decided that women should only wear colors from their seasonal group. Des was a "spring" and actually liked the whole idea but that really didn't matter because she looked great in just about every color under the sun.

Des's parents didn't even ask how we met, which really surprised me. They just commented on how long we'd known each other.

"Two months! That's hardly long enough to think you are in a serious relationship."

More hand squeezing.

They even asked about Tommy, the guy Des had been engaged to, and that was exceedingly awkward.

Des was exasperated. "Well, that's clearly over now, don't you think?"

Aside from the perceived favoritism, they were friendly and nice and very generous with the food and drink, but the tension was palpable. When we got in the car to go home, Des didn't seem to want to talk about it, shrugging it off, instead, with a "I know they love me, but they just don't understand me." But after a few minutes, she did go on to tell me how she felt that they didn't really see or appreciate her. I was sure that wasn't the case but I could also see the pain on her face. That made me even more committed to making her happy. I loved her, I understood her, and I was going to take that pain away.

At that point, the parent introductions were thankfully out of the way, and we were happy to get back to life as we had been deliciously knowing it: classes, studying, grabbing a few beers with some friends...and lots more sex. Life was great.

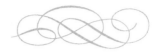

Chapter 3

Des was a "studyaholic" and I liked to lighten things up with trips to the Smith Haven Mall on weekends. The place was lively, the stores were fun to browse around in, and you could get a pretty good slice of pizza at the food court.

We were coming up on Halloween, Des's favorite holiday, and the shops were plastered with all her favorite things - big orange pumpkins, witches on brooms and cutouts of black cats with wild yellow eyes.

"Oh, Robert, look at those jack-o-lanterns! They are soooo great!" she giggled with the enthusiasm of a child. I never much cared for Halloween, but I loved seeing her face light up like that. Des captured all the joy of living with her laugh. It was like oxygen to me, and I breathed it into every pore.

We stopped by a candy stand and I bought her a small chocolate marshmallow pumpkin. She bit into it eagerly. "These are my faves!" she said, and pretty much devoured it in one bite. Des had so many "faves", she embraced her childish enthusiasm for the joys in life.

"And you're my fave!" I said, wrapping her in my arms, and hugging her close and well, I admit it, I put my hand on her behind. She hugged me back and we stayed that way for a long moment before continuing on. Several people walking by gave us that "get a room" look, but we didn't care. We were young, in love and we were happy.

We walked on past a shoe store, a stationery shop and then came up on a jewelry store whose window was filled with watches, necklaces, pins, bracelets, and rings.

Des yanked on my arm.

"Robert - look. That's sooo pretty!"

I turned. Des was eyeing a modest-sized, round diamond ring propped up in a heart-shaped display.

Rings...Uh, oh!

"Isn't it gorgeous?"

It was pretty, I had to admit, and I was sure it carried a pretty price tag. The whole relationship thing was so new and just getting through the parent meetings was enough momentum for me. I hadn't much thought about rings at that point, but I found myself asking, "Wanna try it on - just for fun?"

A huge smile lit Des's face and she bounded into the store. I trailed behind and watched her practically tackle the salesman who was standing near the entrance. She pointed toward the window.

The clerk, a Dabney Coleman look-alike, gave her a big, overly friendly smile, walked quickly to the window and retrieved the ring. When he handed it to her, Des's eyes shone like diamonds themselves.

She glanced at me then put the ring on her finger. I could feel her excitement as she held her hand out and admired it.

It looked great and I had to admit to myself, it had her name on it.

I glanced at Dabney. He glanced back. He was standing, arms crossed, with a satisfied look on his face and visions of a juicy commission no doubt dancing in his head.

By now my heart was thumping big time, but I tried to keep a neutral look on my face. Des looked at me, but I gave her nothing back. She sighed, took off the ring and handed it to the salesman.

He didn't look too happy, either.

We left the store in silence and walked that way for a bit. I nudged Des and tried to elicit a smile. No go. But after a bit, she gave in, smiled and nudged me back.

She had no way of knowing, of course, that my goose was already cooked.

"Come on," I said. "Let's get some ice cream."

She brightened at that, but on our way to the Baskin Robbins stand, we passed a Halloween costume shop where a man dressed as a scarecrow was out in front selling caramel covered apples.

Des stopped in her tracks. "Snoopy, look. Caramel apples! They are one of my favorite things this time of year," she said with such joy while bouncing up and down like a schoolgirl. The way she got excited over the little things in life was captivating.

We headed over to the stand and the smile on her face was priceless.

"Baby, if I buy you an apple will you bounce up and down again for me? You know when you bounce..."

"Robert, you are insatiable," she said with a smirk on her face.

"Can I help you?" the scarecrow asked.

"Yes, one caramel apple please."

"With or without nuts?"

I looked at Des.

"Snoopy, with nuts, it is all about the tart apple, the sugary caramel and salty nuts. It's all the different flavors together which makes it amazing."

"Nuts it is," I responded.

"And for you, sir?" the teenager behind the counter asked.

"Oh, nothing for me," I answered, as I stuck my hand in my pocket and pulled out whatever money I had in there - all two dollars of it.

"What do I owe you?" I asked.

"A dollar."

I reached into my pocket and handed the scarecrow one of the two dollars.

The scarecrow handed her the apple and her eyes lit up at the prospect of biting into the nut-covered, gooey thing...but she stopped, and offered the first bite to me.

"Thanks, Sweetie, but it's not something that's ever interested me. You go on and enjoy it."

"But Robert, you'll love it. I know you will. The contrast between the tartness of the apple and the sweetness of the caramel and the salty crunchiness of the nuts..."

So I took a bite, of course, and she was right – as she usually was when persuading me to try something new. It was delicious and when I got the goo on the corners of my mouth, she reached over and licked it off.

"Gotcha!" she said, with the smile of a conqueror.

"You sure have," I answered. This was the beginning of buying her a caramel apple every October for the rest of our lives together. But at that moment, I had something else I had to do, and I had to make an excuse to escape for a few minutes.

"Think I'd better make a run to the men's room," I said with as straight a face as I could fake. I kissed her on the cheek. "Be right back." I left Des savoring her apple and darted off down the mall, but not for the men's room. I ducked into the jewelry shop. Dabney was showing a middle-aged couple a charm bracelet. He lit up when he saw me: He knew he had a live one.

"I'll be right back with you, folks," he said to his customers.

"So, what can I do for you, young man? Wouldn't have anything to do with that pretty little ring your lovely girlfriend likes so much, would it?"

"That would be a yes," I said. I hesitated for a sec, then looked him straight in the eye. "You gotta hold it for me. Please."

"Of course! Just give me a minute to finish up with those nice folks and we'll do the paperwork."

"Uh, no time right now and, uh, I really don't think we'll need too much paperwork."

I went into my pocket and pulled out my remaining dollar bill. I put it into Dabney's hand.

"Hold the ring for me - please. I'll be back with money every week until it's all paid for."

Dabney looked at the dollar in his hand and started to laugh as he moved his eyes up to look at me.

"This is a prank, right. You're pledging a fraternity."

I looked at him with all the choir boy sincerity I could muster.

"No. Nothing like that. Just hold it for me, OK?"

"Young man, do you really expect me to hold a $1000 ring with a one-dollar deposit?"

"Come on...haven't you ever been in love?"

That must have gotten to him because his face softened.

"I've got a job. I'm good for the money. Really."

He looked at me thoughtfully.

"Well..."

I grabbed his hand and pumped it.

"You'll get every penny of it."

"But..."

"Promise!"

I waved at him and got out of there real fast, but I looked back and saw him walking over to the display and shaking his head as he removed the ring. I breathed a sigh of relief. I had pulled it off. Now all I had to do was come up with the remaining $999.

When I got back to the Halloween store, Des was standing there waiting. The only sign of the apple was a small caramel smudge on the corner or her mouth. I bent over and licked it off. I also moved in for a kiss.

"Thought you didn't like the caramel."

"Ah...it was just my way of sneaking in a kiss."

She laughed.

"So what took you so long? I thought I lost you."

Lost me? I nearly cracked up. I had just signed away my life to her! "There was a line for the john," I said with a straight face.

"Robert, there's never a line for the men's room!"

"I know," I said sounding as shocked as I could about the fictitious line.

It was hard to get away with anything with Des, and I always wondered if she knew. But if she did, she never said anything.

True to my promise to Dabney - he turned out to be a pretty nice guy whose name was actually Charlie - I went back once a month and gave him cash to pay down the ring.

I worked most days after my classes in Mr. DiFalco's grocery store not far from the campus doing whatever needed to be done - clerking, cleaning, delivering orders. I had always worked, ever since I could remember, doing whatever odd jobs I could get... mowing lawns, hauling trash, running errands for people in the neighborhood. I had never wanted to ask my father for spending money.

Mr. DiFalco was a sweet old guy and in addition to paying me minimum wage, which I think was about $3.50 an hour back then, I got to stuff myself with food from the deli counter, so it worked for me.

I socked it away and I finally was able to pay everything off. It was just before Columbus Day of the following year. I remember walking into the mall and the Halloween decorations were up again.

"Hi Robert. How are you doing?" Charlie asked.

"Fine, Charlie...actually better than fine. I'm great!"

"Good to hear."

I handed him an envelope.

"It's all here - everything I still owe you. I'm ready to take that baby home!"

He took the envelope and counted out the money.

"Yup - it's all here, all right...add this $200 to the $800 you've already paid and we're square."

He patted me on the back - something I don't think my father ever did in my entire life.

"I'll be right back with your ring," he said with a huge smile.

I felt so good, at that moment, I wanted to scream for everybody in that fucking mall to hear me. *I got her the ring. I got Desiree Ann Flannery THE ring and soon she'll be mine forever and ever...world without end..."Amen!*

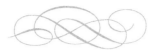

Chapter 4

I had it all planned. I would give Des the ring on her birthday, the following week, but first I had to do the old-fashioned thing and formerly ask Des's father John for her hand in marriage.

I called and asked if I could come up and visit the next day - alone. I suppose her father knew what I had in mind, because he said "sure," and didn't even ask why. It was about seven when I arrived, and they had just finished dinner. Des's dad invited me into the living room and her mom offered me some coffee. I remember not being at all nervous. I guess I was so sure that Des and I were right for each other that I didn't stop to think there might be any impediments.

I stated my business to her father simply. "I think you know by now that I love Desiree...I love her very much. We are great together and I'm pretty sure she wants to spend the rest of her life with me." I looked at him very directly. "I know I definitely want to spend the rest of my life with her."

He cocked his head and gave me a skeptical look. "That's all well and good," he said, "but are you prepared to support her while she finishes school...medical school and all that? She's also planning to get her PhD, as I expect you know."

I nodded my head. "Yes, I know and of course I will support her. I would do anything for your daughter to have what she wants."

"She's a handful," he continued, eyeing me with a half-smile. "Very ambitious - not to mention stubborn."

I nearly broke out laughing because Des had told me that she got her stubbornness from her father and she was so proud to be like him! As for her ambition, I certainly knew about that. It was a given. She would have to be ambitious to even want to deal with all the years of schooling she had ahead of her. Des and I talked constantly about the future...what a great doctor she would be and how I would go on to get my master's in business.

"Yes, sir. I do know and I couldn't be more supportive or more prepared to go the distance."

"And you'll protect her and make her happy?" he asked.

"I'd give up my life for her..."

He looked at me again, for several, very uncomfortable, long seconds, but then he smiled.

"Well, just as long as you know what you're getting yourself into, you have my blessings."

Des's mother joined us and there were smiles all around and that was that. I told the Flannery's that I was planning to give Des a ring on her birthday and invited them to join us for a birthday dinner.

I looked at Des's mother and she nodded at me. I think she had gotten used to the idea of me and had actually grown to like me. "And I think they were both relieved that Des had secured a future husband. It was important to them that their daughter had that part of her life determined at an early age, as they had. Des had told me that they were very traditional in that way.

"We'd be happy to join you for dinner," her dad said.

Secure with the go-ahead, I suggested to Des that we invite her parents to join us for her birthday celebration. I knew she would agree to that. Sharing special times with her parents and always their approval meant so much to her.

We went to a steak place...one of those chains with a big predictable salad bar and the meat that gets served to you either half frozen or charred beyond recognition. The food was almost edible, and we all had an enjoyable evening. When it came time for the check, Des's father didn't reach for it, but that was OK. I think it was part of his wanting to see how prepared I was to take care of his daughter. I was more than ready for it, so it was OK with me.

After dinner we said our goodbyes and Des and I headed back to the dorm. It was a beautiful, cool night, and there were drifts of colored leaves along the path and the streetlamps glowed with that low, yellowish light that made the whole place look kind of magical.

Des liked to step on the leaves and hear the crunchy sound they made.

"Don't you just love it?" she asked as she stepped down into a small mound. "It's such a delicious sound!"

No wonder I loved this girl! Everything made her happy, even the sound of leaves. "And I couldn't wait to make her even happier. I was so anxious to get to her dorm room and give her the ring, I thought I would burst. It seemed that what should have been a five-minute walk took a half hour.

"Hear that?" Des asked looking up at a tree. "It's an owl...a great horned owl, I'll bet."

Only she would know what kind of owl it was. At that point, I couldn't have cared less if there was a god-damned gorilla up there.

"Did you know that they don't migrate like most other birds?"

"No, Des," I laughed, wanting only to migrate to her room so I could give her the ring! "I really didn't know that."

I grabbed her hand. "Hope you liked your birthday dinner, Baby." I said as I pulled her along.

"I absolutely loved it!" she said. "You always do everything to make me happy...like having my parents there. That was wonderful. You know, in many ways I still need to be their little girl and to be fussed over."

"Well, you deserve a fuss - and a big one!"

"And wait till you get a load of the fuss that's about two minutes away...!"

I almost blurted everything out at that point, but I held myself in check.

"Come on," I said, continuing to pull her along. "We're not done celebrating yet!"

She gave me that gorgeous "Des smile" and I could barely stand it for one more minute. I squeezed her hand and we walked into the dorm. Des had her own room, at that point, for which we were both grateful. It gave us the opportunity to be alone together and I actually slept there most nights.

As we got close to her room, Des could see there was something hanging over the door. She started to walk faster and now it was her turn to pull me along. "And when she saw the huge "Happy Birthday" sign I had hung on the door and all the balloons I had put there earlier while she was at the library bouncing around the ceiling like planets drenched in bright Crayola colors, she squealed like little kid. Then she looked around and when she saw the huge arrangement of roses I had put on her desk, she was over the moon.

"Snoopy," she said, as she threw her arms around me. "You are the sweetest, most incredible, most..."

I simply couldn't wait one more minute! I moved her arms from my neck and backed away.

"Come on...sit down. There's something important I need to talk to you about."

She looked at me with the saddest expression I had ever seen.

"Oh, no..." she said, backing away. "All of this was just to make me feel better," she gulped, as she sat down on the edge of her bed. "You're breaking up with me..."

I had to laugh. Only Des would think that. For as happy and light as she was most of the time, she often let dark clouds of fear overcome her. It wouldn't be until years later that I would find out why.

She stared at me for a moment, then started to cry - big, wet sobs. "How can you laugh? I knew it was too good to be true."

She could barely get the words out. "Nothing good ever lasts for me."

A dagger in my heart. What had I done? My big surprise had totally bombed.

"Baby. Don't cry. I never want you to cry."

I had to fix it - fast. I got down on my knees and looked up at her. I was so angry at myself for causing her any kind of pain. "I never thought I would ever feel this way about anyone," I said as I reached up and wiped away the tears that were falling down her cheeks.

She must have believed me because I swear those tears stopped mid-stream.

"You are the most important thing in the world to me. I would give my life for you if I had to."

Now her eyes were teary again, and she put her hand to her mouth.

That's when I reached under the mattress and pulled out the little box. I remember thinking *shit - I forgot to put a ribbon on it,* but that was OK, because unraveling it just would have delayed it that much longer and I didn't think I could have taken one more second.

I opened the box and Desiree looked down at the ring and then looked back at me, her beautiful blue eyes big and wide and staring like a little kid whose letter to Santa somehow had brought exactly what she wanted for Christmas.

"Would you do me the honor of being my wife? I want to spend my entire life with you - always you, only you - now and forever."

Des burst into tears at that point and we held on tightly to each other, neither wanting to let the other go. I will always remember those moments. They were silent, but our hearts spoke volumes.

"Don't you want to put it on?" I asked, after a few moments.

She nodded a big, eager "yes," and I slipped the ring on her finger.

"Oh My God! It's the ring I tried on that day, last year! How..."

"Never mind about the 'how,' Baby. It's the 'why.' It's because I love you so much and there's nothing I wouldn't do for you."

Des grabbed for me again. "I love you, Robert Pardi, Jr. I love you. I love you, I love you."

I knew with every fiber of my being that she did, and that's when I promised to love Desiree Ann Flannery for the rest of her life.

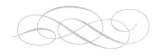

Chapter 5

We moved into an off-campus apartment my senior year, a small, dark studio in the basement of a two-family house. Well, guess it was a three-family house, if you count our bunker. It had one small window, which for sure hadn't been cleaned since the Korean War, an old dresser that tilted way to one side, a small Formica table with two rusty, old chairs and a tiny Pullman kitchen.

It was a dump, but we were thrilled to have our own place. I wasn't especially happy with the kitchen since it had become pretty clear that I was the cook in the family when Des admitted, early on, that she really didn't know how to prepare food. Learning to cook had never been a priority since she had known early on that being a doctor was what mattered most to her.

One day Des very proudly announced that she would make dinner. Ah, a step forward, I thought, but when I came home the place was filled with smoke and the distinct smell of charring.

"What happened, Baby?" I asked.

"I don't know," Des answered innocently. "I put the chicken legs in the broiler, and then this," she said, gesturing to the pathetic pieces of burned chicken that had fallen down through the grates. She had never bothered to put them in a pan.

"Uh, did you defrost them first?" I asked. They were packaged, breaded chicken legs that should have been a cinch to heat up. "And I think you needed to put them in some kind of pan," I said with as straight a face as I could.

Des looked at me so sweetly, so innocently. "Oh, I didn't realize that you had to do that," she said. "I thought you could just cook them."

The look on her face was just so adorable. I couldn't help but to hug her. While she had off-the-charts intelligence, her lack of common sense was sometimes also so off the charts that it was charming. And while my brainiac wife could ace every test at school, she sure as hell couldn't ace the kitchen. So, I was pretty much it. And that was OK with me because I was a pretty good cook. One more reason to be grateful to Grandma Mary. She had taught me to make some pretty mean meatballs.

Tiny kitchen notwithstanding, the place had a really large bed - which practically took up the whole room - and that's what mattered to us. On the day we moved in, the minute we opened the door, I grabbed her hand and we made a beeline for the bare mattress. We rolled around laughing and hugging and feeling that just about everything in our world was right. It had been more than a year, but we still couldn't get enough of each other. Truthfully, I hadn't had all that much experience when Des got a hold of me, but any doubts I had had about myself dissipated. She loved me so much, and never forgot to show me or tell me.

We never told our parents that we were living together. Things were very different back then, and they would have made it pretty rough on us. I don't know who would have been worse - the Irish or the Italians. It was a toss-up that we just decided to avoid.

But we couldn't avoid the issue of money. It was a big concern. What I was earning at the grocery store at that point was not enough, so Des worked too. She tutored students in chemistry, which was pretty amazing because she was able to do it after just reading the textbook once over the summer. But there still wasn't enough money. Des would have to get work in addition to the tutoring, or we would have to stay in the dorms and eke out as many nights together as we could. Neither one of us wanted that.

So Des got a job at a drug store. Aside from the fact that we needed the money, Des loved working there. She enjoyed helping people and answering questions about anything health related.

And she especially liked telling people that she was planning to be a doctor. That always got an "Oh, your parents must be so proud of you!" response. She told me about that with the saddest smile. "Do you think they are proud of me?" she would ask. As smart as Des was, she carried so much self-doubt, so much fear that she was not good enough.

I got the same "your parents must be so proud of you" stuff from some of the little old ladies I waited on in the grocery store, but unfortunately, that had never been the case. I never heard a word of praise out of my father...ever, but I was proud that I was doing what was needed to build a life with Des.

Honestly, I never minded working. In fact, I started working odd jobs at thirteen as a way to decrease my dependency on the old man. Now, however, it was because Des and I needed money for the rent, keeping our old jalopy running, and if she wanted something or needed something, well, I just had to get it for her. And she needed flowers and good food and nights out to have a few beers and let off steam. I loved her so god-damned much I wanted to make her world as wonderful as I could.

Nights out, we used to go to this down-home place that catered mostly to townies in flannel shirts. One night Des and I were at the bar, swigging down a few beers. One of Kenny Rogers' old hits was wafting out of the jukebox. Des was in jeans and a sweater and her hair was lying softly on her shoulders and she looked so off-the-charts gorgeous to me. I just kept staring at her.

"Whaaat?" my innocent angel asked.

"Nothing. It's just that you're the most beautiful, incredible, amazing girl I've ever met."

"Well, then, you're pretty lucky that I picked you!" she said laughing. Then she leaned over and gave me a quick kiss on the cheek.

I pretended to be horrified.

"That's it?" I asked. "I chauffeur you around in our fabulous, old, need-a-screwdriver-to-get-started Volero...buy you one of Bruno's five-star, sausage and pepperoni pizzas with extra cheese...and top it off with drinks at this really exclusive joint, and that's all I get?"

Just about that moment, one of the students from the economics class where I was a teaching assistant walked over to us. I knew right away that this was going to be trouble. Alexis Kramer was a tall, sexy brunette who was always coming on to me in class. I swear I had never done anything to encourage it, except, maybe, just be friendly.

Anyway, she walked over, totally disregarded Des, and focused on me.

"Hey there. Missed you in class today."

She leaned in so close I could feel her breath on my face. I could also feel Des tense up because her knee was leaning heavily against mine.

"Hey, Alexis. Hi. Yeah, something came up."

"However will I understand economics if you don't show up?" she said, looking me up and down. She paused way too long at my crotch.

Uh, oh.

Des put her hand on my thigh and stretched out her fingers. She dug them into my leg.

Uh, oh again.

"Guess you'll just have to study," Des said to her matter-of-factly.

Alexis finally looked at Desiree and then they just stared at each other.

"Oh, Des," I said. "This is "Alexis Kramer. She's in my economics class. You know, the one where I'm a T..."

"Oh, yeah," Des said, without missing a beat. "T."., as in Tits'n ass man."

She glared at Alexis and dug her fingers into my thigh even harder. Des didn't have long nails, but it sure as hell felt like those fingers, alone, could have broken through my flesh. I'm sure I still have the bruise.

"Alexis," I said, "this is my fiancé...Desiree Flannery."

Alexis's face fell so low she needed a crane to pick it back up.

"Oh," she said. "I didn't know you were officially off the market."

"Well, he is," Des piped in. "So buzz off."

I remember smiling because aside from the fact that having two girls fight over me was a huge boost to my ego, I always got a kick when tough talk managed to come out of Des's angelic face. The two so didn't go together. She was sweeter than sweet, but also one of the most determined people you could ever meet. And better not mess with anything that's hers – especially me!

Des and Alexis just kept glaring at each other.

I took a swig of my beer.

"Well, I sure hope you decide to fuh...ooh, I mean not flunk me," Alexis finally said.

Gee-sus. Could she make it any worse?

Alexis gave me one more seductive look for good measure then strutted - and I mean come-and-get-it, ass-wagging, strutted - away.

Des gave her a killer look, took one last swig of beer, and hopped down from her stool. "I'm over this place," she said, and marched off toward the door.

The bartender gave me a big smile. "Nice problem ya got there. Throw one my way if it gets to be too much for you!"

"Feel free to go for the brunette," I said. "The blonde's a keeper - temper and all!"

I put five bucks down on the bar, then rushed off after Des.

At first I was flattered. It was great for my ego, but I didn't see the dark side, at the time, and it turned out to be just the first of many difficult-to-deal-with displays of jealousy.

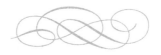

Chapter 6

One day Des and I were at the laundromat. We were both loading up machines and there was this pretty young girl putting things into the washer next to me. I could feel the girl looking at me and I sure as hell could feel Des looking at the girl looking at me.

So the Pretty Young Thing turned to me and said, "Excuse me. Could I borrow some soap?"

Borrow some soap? Who goes to a laundromat and doesn't bring soap? And what about those vending machines filled with one-shot boxes? My antennae should have gone up and I should have turned on the ice, but I didn't have a chance because Des quickly grabbed my arm and switched places with me. Then, in anything but *sotto voce* said, "Honey, be sure to take my stuff out first. You know - your faves - the red lace bra and panties." She let that one ferment for a second then turned to the Pretty Young Thing and gave her a "don't even think about it" smile. It must have worked because the girl didn't look my way again - not even once.

But it was the girls in the economics classes where I was the teaching assistant who really drove Des nuts. As busy as she was with her pre-med studies, one day she took the time to show up in my class.

I was up in the front tackling Keynesian theory and I was really into it. The room was packed with a mix of male and female students, including a few really good-looking girls. If I said I hadn't noticed them I'd be lying, but noticing them and encouraging them were two different things - or at least I thought so.

There were a couple of girls who were clearly more interested in making points with me than in racking up their grades. Or maybe they thought they could kill two birds with one stone. And I have to admit that the stares, the smiles, the crossing and uncrossing of some pretty serious legs were more than mildly distracting.

My mission, nonetheless, was teaching economic theories.

"So the Keynesians believe that markets cannot be counted on to withstand shocks. Prices, wages and other economic markers are not resilient."

John Maynard Keynes was clearly not what the leg-crossers had on their minds, and Alexis, of course, the girl from the bar that ignited the whole jealousy thing, was seated in the first row in a beyond-tight sweater and ridiculously short skirt, and she was slouching to give me a better view of what lurked not so innocently between legs A and B.

"Sound fiscal policies," I continued, "must be employed to create stability."

Frankly, I was a little bit worried about my own stability at that point because I could see Des, at the opposite end of the front row, craning her neck to watch Alexis watching me.

"It's a legacy of economic activism," I went on.

I was sensing disaster and was relieved that the period was coming to an end.

"So for Thursday, I want you to think about what the Reagan administration is doing that reflects Keynesian thinking." The students gathered their stuff and headed for the door. Alexis popped up immediately and corralled me. Des, meanwhile, watched and waited.

"I'm confused about how this differs from the supply and demand theory," Alexis said with a straight face.

I smiled at her - and that was all Des needed. She shot out of her seat like a Cruise missile.

"Couldn't I get you to give me, uh, a private tutorial?" Alexis asked.

"'Kittenish' would be the best way to describe her demeanor - a mix of sexy and coy but fully aware of the powers she had.

This was clearly not how Des wanted the class to end. She grabbed my arm and turned to Alexis.

"I'll give you a little tutorial, sweetie. You wanna talk supply and demand? Well, you can take your demand and shove it, because there sure ain't no supply here. So fuck off!"

That "fuck off" was so loud I thought the campus police would show up any second.

Then Des pulled me to the door and out into the hall. I tried to defend myself as we walked toward the cafeteria.

"Des, honey, I'm not flirting with those girls. It's just..."

"It's just what?" Daggers. "And you were flirting. I saw it."

"Baby, that's just not true." I tried to lighten it up. "Can't you see that I have 'Property of Desiree Flannery' tattooed across my forehead? You're being silly.

Silly. I probably shouldn't have said that because Des hauled off and hit me with a textbook. She was so insecure and there were a few words that I had learned never to use: idiot, stupid and silly being the top three. I had slipped up. I covered my face, pretending to be scared.

"Come on, Des..." I put my arm around her. "You know you are the most important, smartest and most beautiful girl in my life - now and forever."

She looked up at me with those baby blues. "Really?" she asked, as though hearing that had come as a total surprise.

The insecurity that had been surfacing more and more astounded me. This girl had so much going for her, how in Hell could she be so insecure at times? She was actually quite secure when it came to schoolwork. Des was outrageously smart, and she couldn't help but to know it. She almost always got all A's. She even tutored me in organic chemistry – which I loathed – and did it even before she had taken the class herself, which was pretty amazing. It was while I was still in pre-med but itching to switch to economics. One doctor in the family would be enough, as far as I was concerned. I was good in economics and I wanted the kind of lifestyle that a strong business career would support. Des supported that choice. She loved me and wanted me to do whatever it was that made me happy. That she loved me so much made me happiest of all!

Not long after that I graduated and landed a job as Director of Employee Relations in a small investment firm, and rented a small apartment in Dix Hills, not far from my office. Employee relations didn't have much to do with my economics major and it really wasn't what I wanted to do, but it got me in the mix and I figured I could learn a lot. It also paid pretty well, and the money thing was a big factor in my decision. I probably should have held out for a job that would have been a better career move, but I think my judgment was clouded. I was so anxious to build us a solid nest egg.

Des was happy for me that I graduated, of course, but it meant that she had to move back to the dorm, and she wasn't at all happy with that. Neither was I.

"I hate that we're not together," she said. "I miss your smell, your arms around me, your breath on my neck. I miss how you make me feel, Robert. I miss us being together."

"You know it's the same for me, Baby. And this won't be forever," I reassured her.

After being together constantly in school and living together the last year, it was tough on both of us. We lived for weekends when Des would come out to stay with me.

"When we get married, we're going to be together for a hundred years, so you'll be glad when I go off to work in the morning and you can get rid of me!" I said, trying to lighten things up.

She hesitated then said, "I know, but I just hate that you're out in the world and I'm still in school."

"Sweetie, school's a lot more fun than working, and anyway, it's the way it has to be. You've got years of schooling ahead of you - and that's great because when you're done, you're going to set the medical world on fire!"

"I suppose," she said, but she looked at me with such sad eyes.

When Des looked at me that way, I felt awful because I wanted more than anything to make her happy. I knew that if we were married, she would feel so much more grounded, so much more secure. We had targeted the spring of 1990 to get married, and we were in the fall of 1988 at that point, and Des was still nine months away from graduation. But in the weeks prior, I found myself missing her so deeply and thinking more and more that we should move up the wedding date. It made sense to me on every level, so without yet mentioning it to her, I went to St. Andrew's, Des's childhood church, and secured an earlier date - October 15 of the following year.

It was important to Des to be married in that church, so it was important to me. I even booked a great place for the reception. My cousin was the manager of the Astoria Manor, a really nice and quite popular events venue and, aside from the fact that she would do everything possible to make it a perfect evening, she even gave me a break on the price, which I appreciated so much. I had no idea what kind of contribution Des's parents would make. I was excited about the plans and couldn't wait til the end of the evening to tell Des about all the arrangements I had gone ahead and made. I had kept it in a couple of weeks and was bursting to tell her.

We drove the half hour back to her dorm, and as she usually did, Des snuggled close to me the whole time.

"I hate Sunday nights," she said. "I can't wait til we can have them together again, and I can spoil you...you know, bring you treats while we watch tv, make sure you're happy." She gave me one of her wonderful smiles and I found myself wishing it were Sunday night that very moment and we were snuggled in at home together.

"Well, I know your birthday's not for a f
trying to contain my excitement, "but let's

She pulled away, her face lit up in tha·
part curiosity, part impatience - but all be

"I've been thinking," I said as I pullec
move up the wedding date. We don't h
Instead of April,1990, let's get married r
birthday."

"Really?" she asked, wide-eyed.

"Really."

At that moment, I pulled over to the side of the road. There was no way I was NOT going to kiss her.

"Snoopy, what did I do to deserve you?" she practically sang out as she hugged me.

"No, Baby," I answered. "What did I do to deserve *you?*"

"I just hope I make you as happy as you make me."

"Of course you do, I said," and kissed her again and again.

So it was agreed. The wedding would take place in October of the following year. The next thing on the agenda - a conversation with my prospective in-laws. We planned it for the following Sunday afternoon.

Des could not contain her excitement when we arrived at her parents' house. We ushered her mom into the kitchen and the three of us sat down at the table. Des's father was in the next room watching television.

"We decided to move up the wedding," Des said with the same kind of joy she had had the night before when I told her about the plans I had made.

"We've got the date we wanted at St. "Andrew's - Oct. 15 of next year."

"Next year?" her mother asked. "I thought you were planning to wait until the year after."

e changed our minds," Des said, squeezing my hand. of us wants to wait that long."

hen we'll have to talk to Father Mike. He'll want to see you th for counseling." Des's mother was a devout Catholic.

Counseling. Ugh. Des and I looked at each other. We had both forgotten about that.

"It's not a choice," her mother reminded us. Then she called Des's father in and told him the news. He nodded and actually seemed OK with it.

The delicate matter of money had to be broached, but I didn't even have to bring it up. Her parents looked at each other and her father said, "Well, OK, then. We can offer you $5000."

$5000! "Are they kidding? I remember thinking. *It is generous but no way could we do a wedding for $5000 – and certainly not the kind of wedding Desiree should have.*

Well, when we got into the nitty-gritty of it, let's just say we didn't see eye to eye on much of anything about the wedding - who was paying for what, how many people each side would have, the reception venue and even the music. I did my best to keep my cool, but I started to get agitated. I had always had a hard time compromising in general when I was younger. Now, with Des in my life, it was either what she wanted or it was a no-go. Anything that I thought was threatening her happiness became something to fight against.

I could feel Des shifting in her seat. It wasn't going at all the way we had planned. I needed to pull the plug on the discussion quickly.

"Let's think about this all some more and we can talk about it again next weekend," I suggested. "Des has some studying to do for a test, so I want to drive her back to school."

Des looked relieved when I said that. She really didn't have a test the next morning, but both of us needed to leave – and to leave, then. I pretty much knew what I was going to do going for-ward, but at that moment, I just had to get us out of there.

"Come on Baby," I said. "Let's get you back to school." I grabbed her hand and tugged. Des and I were completely on the same page about it. We said our goodbyes and left.

"It'll all be fine, honey," I said as we drove back to Stony Brook.

"I know it will, Robert" Des said. "I have never understood how,

but you always make everything fine. I think you can even change the weather for me. You're not a warlock or some weird wizard, are you?" she joked and snuggled against me as we drove.

Truth was, I had expected Des's parents to pay for the wedding, as was the custom, but in a way, I was glad that it turned out that way because I didn't want anyone controlling our lives - not Des's family or mine, for that matter. In fact, my Mom and I had already had a few "discussions" by that point. So the next day I went to the bank and took out a loan for $10,000. That, added to the $8000 I had in my bank account, would give us enough to have a really nice wedding - and one that we, ourselves, would be in charge of.

The day after that, I drove back out to her parent's house and told them that Des and I would take care of everything and while they were both surprised, I think by my taking the financial reins it showed them - especially Des's father - that I really was capable of taking care of their daughter. They seemed to respect me more after that.

So Des and I ran the whole thing. We had the big church wedding followed by a nice reception. We chose the invitations, picked the music, flowers and photographer...well, actually, Des did a lot of the sourcing and gave me the parameters for making the final choices. I even did the seating, taking care to keep the Capulets nicely distanced from the Montagues. We totally agreed about that! Desiree was storybook beautiful and when I close my eyes, I can still see her perfectly - a fairytale princess with that gorgeous smile, her long, blonde hair falling in big curls and a Jessica Mc-Clintock wedding gown that would rival any ever worn by a real-life princess. She was *my* princess and when we danced our first dance as Mr. and Mrs. Robert Pardi, Jr., I knew I was the luckiest guy who had ever walked on God's earth.

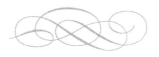

Chapter 7

When Des and I wanted to relax and talk about life, stresses at school or our dreams for the future, we often went to the beach near Port Jefferson on Long Island, where we'd take long walks on the sand, look out at the sea, and think about all the places we wanted to visit. Our old Valero was still alive and kicking and it had large seats in both front and back. Sometimes at night we would take advantage of the big back seat and make love. God knows what would have happened if a cop or anybody, for that matter, had come along, but we were lucky because no one ever saw us.

We liked to drive around the Island and look at the big mansions and occasionally, if we found one under construction, we'd go in and pretend what it would be like to be really rich.

"I could get used to this!" Des would say.

"Hey," I would tease. "You're supposed to be the do-gooder in this group. Don't tell me you're becoming Republican!"

"Never!" she laughed.

This was before the wedding and of course we talked about what our lives would be like after we were married.

"It will be more perfect than ever," Des said, "especially if we start things off away from all the drama of our families."

It was such a beautiful evening and Des was nibbling on my ear and to be honest, I really didn't think about what that meant, but we were so in heaven, I remember saying "sure."

She looked at me with those baby blues and cocked her head. "Snoopy," she cooed, "after we get married, let's move to Arizona."

"Arizona? Sure, Baby. I'll just fire up the private jet!" I joked. We had been to Arizona a couple of times and had really liked it. On both of those trips, Des had found it very tranquil, and talked about how much fun it would be to live there.

"Sure it would be fun," I agreed, "but we don't have much of a nest egg to fall back on. We'd be taking quite a risk."

"Well, I took a risk on you, didn't I?" She said that with such a straight face, before nuzzling into me with a big smile, I caught my breath for a second or two.

Des made risk-taking seem like the meaning of life...to run after a dream, sometimes not fully thinking it through but always losing herself in the joy of the pursuit. She believed that to live fully, not only did you have to take risks, you had to experience joy in doing it.

I believed in risk-taking, too – but calculated risk taking, and sometimes we would not be on the same page about things. Des, however, found so much joy in taking new paths, in being able to throw caution to the winds.

"Snoopy, you know, we only live once," was one of her favorite lines to support her argument to take a risk.

I marveled at it. It seemed to be in direct competition with her extraordinary, razor-sharp mind, but it was who she was and I learned so much from her about living life and loving it. She was a beautiful bundle of extraordinarily captivating contrasts.

"Arizona...let's do it!" she said. "University of Arizona med school is world-class, and it's in Tucson." There was so much enthusiasm in her voice, there was no way I could veto the idea. "We could go straight from our honeymoon. That way we can enjoy being together and learn to be a team, without the pulls and the family dynamics. "And you know how much I love the desert," she whispered in my ear, making sure that her tongue tickled it to seal the deal. "It's so calming."

Des loved the desert and the ocean and the mountains and the lakes and dogs and cats and horses and babies and old people. There wasn't much that girl didn't love, and that was great, just as long as she loved me.

While at the time I just thought it was part of her fun-loving nature, I had no idea how important that philosophy would be to her - to both of us - in later years, or how grateful I would be that she showed me that path, and how it permeated my soul and became one of my core values.

When I thought about moving to Arizona for a while, it really did seem to be a good idea. Des was right about learning to be husband and wife without anyone else interfering - and we expected plenty of that from both sets of parents. So I agreed that after our honeymoon we would continue on to Arizona, where we would plan to spend at least six months before plunging into the real world.

As it turned out, Des decided not to apply to medical school until the following semester. That came as a huge surprise because I knew she was so eager to get started on her path to being a physician, but she wanted us to be able to have time together before settling into the pressure of all that studying and all those bills - and to be honest, I was happy she made that decision. It was a gift to our relationship - a gift to me. It would also give her time to get her grant applications in order. Her grades had always been so good, she was confident the grants would come through.

She subsequently did go on to get those grants from the NIH, which gave her a modest annual stipend and paid for her eight years of schooling - two years of medical school followed by a PhD program in physiology and biophysics, then the final two years of med school. But that certainly would not be the end of it. Her future would include an internship and then a residency and who knew what else? It would be an awfully long haul, so I really liked the idea of having her all to myself for a few months before *that* schedule kicked in.

We chose Daytona Beach, Florida for our honeymoon. At that point, we had traded up to a black Nissan, and as we zoomed down I-95 to Daytona Beach, we listened to the radio – songs like Taylor Dane's "I'll Always Love You," which was our wedding song, and Bette Midler's "Wind Beneath my Wings." The popular songs of the moment seemed to be written just for us. Des always loved long drives. I would talk and she would sing. She had a really good voice and I always thought had she not been so committed to being a doctor, she might have gone for a career in music. Whenever a song by her favorite group Heart came on, that was my signal to keep quiet and let her just sing out. Well, that afternoon she was in top voice and when Heart sang "What About Love, don't let it slip away. What about love, I only want to share it with you," there was no way I could ever be happier than I was in that moment. Des was singing to me and we were married and together and we had our whole long future ahead of us.

We drove for nearly 21 hours straight through, with just food and comfort stops. We luxuriated in the sun, took long walks on the beach, ate lobster nearly every night, and spent an inordinate amount of time in the room. Hey, it was our honeymoon and we did the tradition proud.

After 10 days, we were in the car again, whooping it up, heading west on Route 64. We arrived in Scottsdale, Arizona two days later, and went immediately to the mall. Oh, did I forget to include shopping in that list of things that Des loved? For a girl with a beyond-serious brain and plans for an important career, shoes and bags and sweaters and skirts and lip gloss and hair stuff were all right up there in that part of her cerebrum not dedicated to her future as a world-class physician. Sometimes that "girly-girl" stuff made no sense to me at all, but I did like seeing her have whatever she wanted, and she loved seeing me get new things for myself.

We had already bought new boots and some western shirts when a pet shop loomed just ahead. If ever alarms should have immediately gone off in every part of my body, it was then, but by the time all my nerve endings started to scream, it was too late. Desiree was already gushing over a caramel-colored Pomeranian puppy in the window.

"Oh my God. Robert, look at him! He's a teddy bear!"

God, he *was* cute - but no way! "Sweetie, remember," I said, "no real-world responsibilities right now. Nothing to tie us down."

"But, Snoopy - he's soooooooo cute!"

"Yeah, and, sooooooooo expensive, I'm sure!" I was already in hock to the bank for the wedding and there would be tons more on my credit card for the honeymoon and our expenses in Arizona. Cute as this little guy was, I didn't need to add on whatever it would cost to buy him, not to mention vet fees and food and grooming and on and on.

Well, I didn't win that one - not that I won many. In less than a half hour we were in the car...Desiree, me and the pedigreed fluff ball who was in her lap and licking her face, big time. Lucky dog! Now it was my turn to be jealous.

That little guy cost $1000. A thousand dollars! Absolutely and totally insane, but it made Des happy, so it was worth every penny. We named him Dollar$ and spelled his name with a dollar sign to remind us just how crazy we really were.

But Dollar$ was just the beginning of our spending spree. There were the restaurants and more clothes and since we were in the southwest, we had to have a jeep, of course, so we went one better and bought an Izuzu Amigo. That one was my big indulgence. We used to drive out into the dessert and just lie back and look at the stars, which was an incredible experience and something we never could have done in New York City.

"Look how amazing they are!" she often said. "I just wish I could reach out and grab one."

I totally understood that. The sky was magical.

The holidays were coming and I wanted to be sure we had a special Christmas - our first as a married couple. Des was always like a little girl during the holidays and being able to feel that joy was as much a part of her as was her determination to be an amazing doctor. My greatest joy was to see that joy in her, and our star-watching trips gave me an idea. When Christmas arrived - complete with paper mâché snowmen and Arizona cactus plants sporting jolly Santa hats - I surprised Des with a huge box.

"Dollar$, what did daddy get me?" she asked, all smiles. She eagerly opened the box and saw the rolled-up document inside.

"What is it Robert? Did you make so much money without telling me that you bought me a medical degree?"

"No need for that. You're going to get that all on your own. But you're my special star, Baby and you will forever be the force that guides my life," I said. "Now there's a star that for all eternity will be named 'Desiree.' This certificate authenticates it."

Des loved unconventional gifts and this one was clearly up there. She jumped up on me and hugged me as tightly as she could and then Dollar$ jumped on both of us and started barking. Then, in seconds, our clothes came off and Dollar$ knew it was time for him to move to the other end of the room. We fell asleep on the floor that night and while we had no fireplace from which to hang stockings and a strange-looking Christmas tree, it was a beyond perfect Christmas.

Des was thrilled with her star and she kept that certificate framed and on the wall of every apartment we ever lived in. It cost me a modest amount, but it made her so happy, and even though we were in the hole, I would have spent thousands to get it for her.

But the hole continued to get deeper. While I could budget and invest with the best of them, when it came to Des, I was blinded by her smile and my desire to make her happy, whatever the cost.

Even though we both got jobs to fund our little adventure - Des as an assistant at a local product-testing laboratory and I as a rep for a Long Island broker who paid me a moderate salary to find wealthy retired clients in Arizona - we found it harder and harder to make ends meet. Our money finally ran out, and we had to go home. The fact that we had to return east wasn't so bad, but with no money and nowhere to live, we were forced to live with Des's parents. I think my mother would have liked us to stay with her. That way she could have her baby boy back, but we ended up opting for Des's folks.

We were expected to help around the house, of course, and kick in for food, and that certainly seemed fair, but Des wasn't thrilled to be back home - especially as a married woman - and I, sure as hell, wasn't happy about being there. I never felt welcome, or at ease or part of the family. I also didn't like some of the conversations.

One night, for example, Des's father jabbed at her about med school. He put down a fork full of pot roast long enough to ask, "And how's the job of yours? I'm sure you're doing important work at the lab, but I thought you'd be in medical school by now."

"Assisting an important scientist with his experiments is a great education," Des answered. "Textbooks are one thing, but the real stuff happens in the lab! I'm learning an awful lot, and it will only help me in the future. Besides, I can't think of a better way to spend my time while I apply for the MD/PhD program."

I felt she shouldn't have had to defend herself in this way, because she was on such a clear path when it came to her medical and scientific education. Looking back, I realize that it was just her father's wanting everything to go well for her. We were so young, and he had her best interests at heart. Des always felt stung, however. If she had voiced her feelings and cleared the air, it would have been so much better, all around.

Not long after that, we got the hell out of there and rented our own apartment. I had gotten a pretty good job at a small investment firm in the city and I felt my career focus was back on track. We found a six-story walk-up on New York's upper east side. It was a small studio with ordinary white walls, and we furnished it with really inexpensive furniture - the kind you buy raw and have to paint yourself, but it was bright and sunny and had a great Murphy bed. And we had our privacy...well, if you're not counting Dollar$ wanting to get in on everything, that is!

Des was now working as a lab tech at Mount Sinai Hospital. She really liked being there and loved the work she was doing. As for me, the lifestyle that would be possible by making it big on Wall Street was what motivated me, and that meant getting a graduate degree from a really good school. My first choice was Columbia, and I was accepted in the Executive MBA program, which allowed me to work professionally four days and week and attend classes on the fifth and sixth. My new boss was good with that. At last, things were going great. We were happy.

The firm where I landed a job was a small company in midtown Manhattan. Actually, it was just the owner and me, but the guy I replaced had gone on to bigger and better things, and I was hoping I would follow in his footsteps. The boss, 60ish, scrawny and scraggly looking, kept his trousers up with old suspenders and made a habit of keeping a fat, chewed-over cigar in his mouth, but I learned a lot from him and he treated me like a son which, considering my history, made me appreciate him on several levels. I welcomed the relationship, and the opportunity.

Desiree, on the other hand, was getting crazed because she had so many years of school ahead of her and I was already out in the real world. She hated when I worked late and we didn't get to have dinner together. And, yes - of course - she was jealous of all the fabulous women out there she thought were after me. Well, I'm here to tell you my bevy of beauties, in fact, consisted mostly of little old ladies who needed help with retirement allocations. Occasionally, I'm loathe to admit, one of them would take a shine to me and it took some careful finessing on my part. The boss was all for it because this clientele was his firm's meat and potatoes and he encouraged me to take the women out to lunch or dinner on the firm. "Those old broads like to be romanced!" he would say. Back then, a certain kind of man liked to refer to women as "broads." Today they are skewered for language like that – justifiably!

I remember coming home one night about 10:30, really anxious to see Des, and I took the six flights two stairs at a time. I put my key in the door and when I opened it, the apartment was dark, but I could see her curled up in a chair by the window.

"Sweetie, what are you doing sitting in the dark?" I asked as I flipped on the light switch.

She looked up and I could see her face was red and swollen from crying. I rushed over to her.

"Baby...what's wrong?"

"I called your office around 5:30 and they said you had just left for dinner - with a woman."

Thinking about the client I had just eaten with - an overweight, overly made-up retiree, I started to laugh.

"It's not funny, Robert!"

"First of all," I said, kneeling down, "you have to see this woman! Bitter, rude, corpulent, would be putting it mildly, 70-ish and even if I was the last man on earth... Regardless Baby, I have you, how in the world could I ever give up the best for something, well in this case, at the bottom of the cesspool?"

Des stared at me for a few seconds and then came back with, "And what about Nicole, that girl at the gym? I see how she looks at you!"

I had gotten Des to start going to the gym with me and like everything else she tackled, she took to it from the get-go and with my coaching was doing the Nautilus like a champ.

I had barely been aware that there were other women at the gym, let alone anyplace else, and Des's jealousy was becoming a problem - a big one. I was busting my chops at school and at work and I couldn't possibly have been more in love with her than I was. The last thing I had on my mind was cheating, with clients, Nicole from the gym or anyone else. I was at a loss to figure out why she had a jealousy problem - which seemed to be getting worse as time went by - except that it had begun to be pretty clear that it had a lot to do with her self-esteem. The girl was brilliant and beautiful. She had every confidence in her intellectual capabilities, but on an emotional level, she never thought she was enough, no matter how often I reassured her.

"Baby, this distrust stuff has got to stop. Nicole is just a friend and besides, everyone at the gym sees how in love with you I am."

She began to cry and then I felt terrible.

"I'm out there trying to make a living - a future for us. And you need to know - there are women out there –all kinds of women, and there always will be. Doesn't mean I'm interested now or will ever be. You've got to know that, believe that, or we're not going to make it."

"That's just it," she said. "You're out there in the world, and I've got years of school ahead of me. It just doesn't match up." She sighed, then looked at me sadly. "I think I need to leave."

What! "Leave? What are you talking about?"

Where the hell did this come from? I was blindsided. I pulled Des to her feet and wrapped my arms around her. "Baby, we're just beginning!"

It was clear to me that something very positive had to happen very soon that would make Des feel better about herself, or we would implode. She had to get her medical career going.

"Here's what has to happen now," I said sternly. "It's time for you to ditch that job of yours and start medical school. The dream begins today - and not a minute later."

Des started to smile. She could do that - be sadder than sad or mad as hell one minute then bubbly and happy the next. Not me. I enjoyed some good brooding time.

Then she looked up at me, all clear-eyed now. "You're right, Robert."

So, over the next few weeks, she got back on track, studied for her MCATS, the medical school admissions tests, took the exams... and we waited. There was no doubt in my mind that she would sail through with top grades. She always did. But to help her feel more confident - and special - the night before the exam I took her to a hotel on Long Island and helped her study. The fact that we were in a hot tub made it a lot more fun, and all the laughing we did helped diffuse her anxiety.

The day of the test, I came to pick her up with Dollar$ in one hand and roses in the other.

"I haven't passed yet, Robert," she protested. But Dollar$ and I were sure that she had and one night after dinner, a few months later, she casually reached down to the table where some mail was piled, picked up some envelopes and without so much as blinking an eye said, "I got into Mass General." "And then with a smile added, "and Brigham and Women's."

I couldn't believe how nonchalantly she just let those names roll off her tongue.

"Brigham and Women's. My God, Des - that's Harvard!"

The smile got bigger.

"And Mount Sinai, too."

"And Mount Sinai, too," I mimicked. "You devil!"

Now I had her laughing.

"Baby, you're amazing! But it'll be Harvard, won't it?"

"Are you kidding? It'll be Mount Sinai. Do you think I'm going to leave you alone in New York with all your women?"

She was only half kidding.

"And did you think I would ever let you go to Boston alone?" I asked. "I can always get something up there."

"No, Robert, all jokes aside. We are a team and we will always be a team and if I can pursue my dream in a place that offers you the most opportunity, then there is no choice. I know you put me and my career first above yourself." She reached for my hand. "Mount Sinai offers me a lot of opportunities, and when I finish, it will be your turn to come first."

Desiree taught me that a relationship is not one person winning and the other losing. It's the pursuit of common goals and she was right - but for me, she came first. ALWAYS.

She shook her head and said "Mount Sinai" and the choice was made - just like that. "And then, like there had been no tears and no scene and no life plans re-sorted, Des looked at me all innocent like and asked, "So what are you going to make me for dinner?"

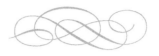

Chapter 8

Things were really good after that. Our lives were full, if not a bit chaotic. Des started med school, and I continued working while going for my MBA. We were everybody's idea of a fun New York couple...the walkup apartment, the dog, the crazy neighbors, including Lola across the hall, a would-be actress and dancer who waited tables at a nearby pub.

One night, Des and I had been out for a few beers and I chased her up the stairs and pinned her against the door. Lola emerged from her apartment, looked at us and shook her head.

"Don't give him too much lovin', Des. Spoils 'em."

"Too late for that!" Des said. "Trust me, he's already spoiled rotten!"

We both laughed at that one because Des and I both knew who had spoiled whom!

"So how are the auditions coming?" Des asked.

Lola gave us her big show-business smile. "Well, I had two callbacks on A Funny Thing, and one on Chicago." She did a quick soft-shoe and curtsied. "Meanwhile," she continued, "I'm still waiting tables at Friday's. And I'd better hustle." She glanced at her watch. "I'm late. One more time and they'll fire my ass!"

"Don't worry, Lola," Des said. "Your big break will come. It's bound to happen!" She jabbed me in the side. "Isn't it, sweetie?"

"Uh, yeah. For sure," I said, hoping I sounded convincing.

Lola started down the stairs, then turned around, with a big smile.

"And when it does happen, you guys will be in the front row - on me!"

"Imagine trying to make it on Broadway," I said as we walked into our apartment. Then I asked, "Aren't you glad you decided to be a doctor and not a dancer?" The minute that came out of my mouth I knew it had been a huge mistake.

Des whirled around. "Excuse me! Like med school is nothing?"

"Des - I didn't mean it like that!"

"Then how did you mean it? You think that what I'm doing is easy?"

"No. Of course I don't. It's just that you're so damned smart, it's easy for you."

"Thanks, but that doesn't mean I don't need support."

And she was right. I understand, now, that even the most competent people need support. I was glad she verbalized it, but as it turned out, there was more to the story than not feeling supported - much more - and I didn't find out about it until the nightmares started to come.

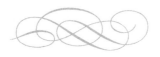

Chapter 9

Since the beginning of our relationship, Des nearly always had slept very peacefully, mostly curled up in my arms. Of late, however, her sleep had become troubled. She groaned, mumbled, and thrashed around quite a bit, and when the mumbling became louder, it was clear she was having nightmares. When I nudged her, she'd stop and fall back to sleep. I asked her about it, of course, but she always said she didn't remember having any bad dreams.

Then, at one point several nights going, she kept repeating "No, Eric... Stop!" Eric, please! No...no!"

"Baby – what's wrong?" I asked, shaking her.

She continued to toss. "No, Eric. You can't!"

"Wake up, Des. You're having another nightmare."

Her eyes popped open. She stared at me for a long moment. Her breathing was labored.

"Who's Eric, Des? You've been calling his name - well, screaming it, actually."

"Uh, what? What do you mean?"

"Des, you were screaming about somebody named Eric, telling him to stop."

She looked at me with a blank expression.

"Who is he?" I asked.

She hesitated, then said, "Oh...nobody."

"Sure sounded like somebody to me, and what was he doing?"

"I said it was nobody," she snapped. "And it's nothing, so drop it - OK?" She rolled over.

Well, it was pretty damn clear to me that this Eric, whoever he was, was hardly nobody and whatever it was, was hardly nothing.

Then she turned to me and, sweet as pie, thanked me for waking her out of it. "I'm better now. Really." She kissed me on the cheek. "Let's go back to sleep. See you in the morning."

She turned over again, burrowed down into her pillow, and drifted off.

No such luck for me. I was no shrink, but I didn't have to be Sigmund Fucking Freud all these years to know that Des had some real issues. Maybe the nightmares meant she was finally coming to grips with them.

But who the hell was Eric? I knew about that guy she was engaged to when she met me, but I thought his name was Tommy. She had resisted talking about him, and since I had clearly won the race, it didn't seem to matter much. Maybe it should have...

The next morning Des was bright and cheerful and totally dismissive of the night before. When I asked if she wanted to talk about it, I got a big smile, a kiss and a "Have a good day."

I should have pressed her...but I didn't. She could do that to me - have one of these episodes or a knock-down drag out and then be all sweetness and light and I would just let it go. Guess I was so busy worrying about *her* head, I wasn't looking at mine.

By now, Des had done two years in med school and had moved on to working on her PhD in physiology and biophysics at The City University of New York at Mount Sinai. She was really into her studies, and I loved seeing her that way. As insecure as she could be in our relationship, the exact opposite was true with her work. She had all the confidence in the world about her academic abilities. She was incredibly smart, and she knew it.

I got my MBA, meanwhile, and moved on to a bigger job at an investment house, where I was a senior equity research analyst. I was finally growing and I felt good about it.

Although Des was acing her way to her PhD, she still wasn't making much progress on an emotional level. We had some nasty fights, like the time we were having a perfectly nice evening and, out of nowhere, she exploded.

It was a warm, late spring night. Des and I were walking the dog down a quiet side street in our neighborhood. Dollar$ spotted a fire hydrant and forged ahead to check it out. The hydrant was surrounded by some messy garbage and I wasn't crazy about him doing his business there, so I yanked him away.

"Not that one, boy. It's filthy!"

Then, out of the clear blue, Des screamed at me. "It's not bad enough that you tell me what I can and cannot do. Now you're bossing him around."

What?

"What the hell are you talking about?"

"You're always trying to control me."

Control her?

"Have you completely lost your mind?" I asked.

And she came back with, "Are you calling me crazy?"

And here we go again...

"Did I say anything about being crazy?"

Now I was getting pissed. "I think all those hours studying have gotten to you. You need a break."

Well, that was just the intro she needed.

She glared at me. "You're absolutely right about needing a break. What I need a break from is you - I want out!"

I couldn't believe she actually said that, and I guess my pride was wounded because I found myself saying, "You know, I think I'm the one who needs a break. I've had it with your tantrums. You are my first and last thought every fucking day. No, this is it. It's time for me to move out and on!"

Des just looked at me.

The pain was great and I couldn't believe what I said next, but I just couldn't take it anymore. The joy we had was bleeding away, and something radical had to happen. I'm not sure exactly what I was thinking at that moment, but this time she had pressed my buttons one time too many.

"I'm leaving," I said firmly. "And don't expect me to come back."

Des had threatened to leave before, many times during her jealous outbursts over the years. I always knew she was bluffing, being defensive, and needing me to confirm my love for her, so I just took it. But I remember telling her that, if I ever left, I would never be back. I did have *some* pride.

"Here," I said, handing Dollar$' leash to her. "Take your damn dog. See if it's enough love for you."

I took a few steps, my heart beating wildly, then turned back around.

"You know, there are a lot of women out there who would like my kind of, uh, control. I'm leaving, and I won't be back." And with that, I walked away.

The dog starting barking and I could hear Des say, "No, Dollar$. Let him go. He'll be back."

At that moment, I was so pissed, I had no intention of going back. It was painful - incredibly painful. I loved her, but I just couldn't take any more of the insanity. Dollar$ was barking loudly, but as I walked to the end of the block, I could hardly hear him, my heart was beating with such force that I could hear the beat echoing in my ears. Without looking back, I rounded the corner and with a few more steps was at Jimmy's, one of our favorite places, where I could numb the pain with a few beers.

I was just yards away, so on some level I must have known that it wouldn't take too much to find me - assuming she wanted to find me - and in a little while, I felt a tap on my shoulder. There she was, sweet as an angel, tote bag over her shoulder with Dollar$' little head sticking out of it.

"I'm so sorry, Robert. Please forgive me."

I was still pissed and I tried my best not to turn toward her.

"I love you so much...too much. Please don't leave me."

She leaned into my back and I could feel the tears falling. Those tears were always my weakness.

I turned to face her. "And you know how much I love you, Des, but I can't take this anymore. I just can't. Things have got to change. You know I would give my life for you, why don't you see that?"

She looked so sad, so forlorn. Then I felt guilty, and I hated myself. *How fucked up was this?*

"Come on," I said. "Let's see what we can do to fix this."

Des sat down on the stool next to me, and I signaled the bartender.

"Heineken for my wife, please."

She was still crying. I dabbed at her tears with my fingers. Every last bit of my resolve had dissipated.

Des reached for me and hugged me close, and we stayed that way for a long time.

"Let's go home," I said. "We've got lots to talk about."

We left, holding hands, and didn't say all that much as we watched Dollar$ bound ahead in front of us. When we got home, we settled in on the sofa and talked for hours. The pain that Des had been carrying around for as long as she could remember had finally erupted. Now was the time to talk about it.

As smart as Des knew she was, she still never felt that she was enough. Much of her insecurity seemed to boil down to the way she perceived her parents felt about her, and how she somehow felt in competition with her mother who, as she explained to me, mentioned more than once that her own grades in nursing school had been excellent. She described it as feeling "less than" and "being pushed, rather than coddled." She knew both her parents loved her, it was so obvious to me, but Des had developed this negative perspective, harboring a deep feeling that she was never enough.

Her mother was, indeed, a very smart woman and only eighteen years her senior and even though it was clearly obvious how much her parents loved her and did their best for her, at that moment, what I felt was rage. It was so painful to see my brilliant, high-achieving wife regress to a seven-year-old child right in front of me. I just couldn't understand where this all originated from. I felt inadequate because I wanted to, but I didn't know how to fix it for her. It was devastating to me to see Des in pain that way, as she explained to me how she felt.

"You've got to get this all out, Baby. It's been coming out in your dreams. I want so much for you to feel better...to feel good."

She looked at me with such sadness. I pulled her close.

"I am here for you now, and will always be here for you, to protect you and love you. I hope you know that."

She nodded and nestled in closer, her tears still falling.

Things were slowly starting to make sense...the jealousy and the threatening to leave. She was so sure she was not enough, so sure I would leave her, she wanted to preempt me and do the leaving herself. It would hurt less that way.

Intellectually, she knew all the answers. Internalizing them on an emotional level was another story. Most of it made sense to me, but the missing piece fell into place when she finally told me about Eric.

It was practically dawn that same night. She was lying in my arms and I think we both just wanted to drift off that way, but we were almost there, so I had to press on.

"There's one more thing I need to ask you about...Eric. Who's Eric?"

"Who?"

"Eric. You're still yelling 'Eric' in your sleep."

I felt her whole body stiffen.

"I...I can't talk about it."

"Des, we've got to clear the air on this. There's still something you're holding back and obviously it's important."

She tried to avert my eyes.

"Come on. We're on a roll."

She looked at me for a long moment. Tears gathered in the corner of her eyes. She finally shook her head in resignation. Whatever it was that was gnawing at her had to come out, and this was the moment for it.

She sighed deeply, then slowly started to talk. "Eric...uh...well, he was this kid who lived down the street. I'd known him forever. He was about three years older than me and we were friends. I really liked him, but I didn't like the kids he hung out with. They were loud and had really dirty mouths, and I was never comfortable being around them." She wiped the tears away with her hand. "A couple of them were real smart asses who used to make nasty remarks when they saw me...especially about my breasts. I was only thirteen, but they were already big and they would yell at me, things like...'Yo jugs, need a chest rub?' and 'Don't be shy. You know you'd like it.' Remarks like that. And then they would all crack up. It made me feel awful."

Her voice was sad, and I knew that this story was not going to have a happy ending. She moved to face me and sat cross-legged. I tried reaching for her hand, but she pulled back.

"One afternoon, I was coming home from school and Eric was waiting in front of my house. He didn't have his creepy friends with him which I was glad about that. He often used to come in, and we would grab a snack, go up to my room, and listen to music. We both loved listening to music, and it was fun just to hang out. I never thought much about being alone with Eric and even sitting on my bed with him. I really liked him. It had always been so innocent. I was only thirteen.

"He kissed me and it was so sweet. We kissed for a while but then he pushed me down on the bed and started moving his hands all over me. I tried to get up, but he wouldn't let me up. I remember having the worst feeling in the pit of my stomach. What was he doing? I pleaded with him to let me go but that didn't seem to matter to him. He was supposed to be my friend, to care about me. He covered my mouth so I couldn't speak and before I knew it, she gulped. Robert, she hesitated, Robert, he was so much bigger than me, so much stronger, and...."

Des stopped mid-sentence and looked at me. I tried again to reach for her hand, but again she pulled back. I knew where this was going and said, "Baby, you don't have to say anything else if you don't want to. We can stop here."

"No, I have to Robert. I have to!"

Her face became so red, I could see the rage in her face and then she said, "He raped me, Robert. He raped me...this boy I had known since I was a little kid." Her eyes welled up with tears. I couldn't believe he would disrespect me that way."

"When he was finished, he just got up and left. Didn't even say anything to me. Nothing. Not one word. I just stayed in my room, immobile, staring at the wall. I don't know how long I sat there. Finally, I got up and went into the shower and made the water hotter and hotter until it practically scalded me, hoping to wash the experience away. After that, I did everything I could to stay as far away from him as possible. I never spoke to him again - and I never told anyone - until now."

There's no adequate way to describe how I felt at that moment. White hot anger, horror, a thirst for vengeance, but mostly love, love for this precious girl to whom this never should have happened. I reached for her hand a third time and she cautiously let me.

"I didn't even tell my mother. I suppose I should have, but I was so ashamed...so ashamed that I had lost my virginity like that. I also didn't want anyone to look at me like I was broken or damaged. So I just kept it in." She swallowed hard. "I swear it wasn't my fault. I know I should have bit his hand or kicked him in his balls, but I just felt paralyzed, like I was out of my own body. I swear it wasn't my fault."

The tears were streaming down Des's face now, and as long as I live, I will never forget that look. I put my arms around her and held her like a child. "Of course it wasn't your fault!"

Where is that guy now? I'd like to get my hands on him.

"It's all OK, Baby," I said. "We're together and I will always protect you. I will be your warrior forever. Everything is OK now."

She cried and cried until finally, there were no tears left.

Following the assault, she explained, the experience took its toll. She became ashamed of who she was and the very womanly figure she was developing and resorted to wearing baggy clothes to hide it.

"My breasts were just so big...too big, and I felt I had to cover them. They made me feel ashamed. They were why he came after me in the first place." She then explained that as she grew further into her teens, she started to dress and act provocatively, which just left her feeling ashamed and magnifying her already serious lack of self-respect.

"Then I started to learn that my body was a way...I don't know...a way to manipulate guys. It was messed up. My whole sexuality was messed up until we met and you treated me as a person." She said that with such sadness that I felt my own eyes well up.

"Shush...Baby. You're safe, now," I said. "All of those awful things are in the past. I'm here. It's you and me, just you and me. And you will never have to be ashamed of anything with me – ever. I love you."

It all became clear to me – the nightmares, the insecurities, her feeling of not being enough, and the jealousy. I loved her more in that moment than I thought I was ever capable of loving anyone. I knew that nothing I could ever do would make up for all the pain she had had, but I sure as hell was going to try. I would do anything and everything for this precious girl and would never allow anything bad to happen to her ever again, of that I was sure.

Some say that keeping a marriage together in the seventh year is a challenge. Seven-year-itch, it's called. Well, for us, it was a new beginning. We were one person, after that.

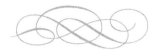

Chapter 10

Years later in med school, as busy as she was, Des managed to find time to volunteer for The New York Help Line, providing emotional and moral support for anonymous callers in crisis. When I look back, I marvel at how she was able to fit it all in but that was who she was...caring about others and doing whatever she could, whenever she could to make lives better. She spent hours on the phone, listening to people in trouble and counseling them, making use of all the self-help books she had read, all she had learned as a psych major in college, and certainly her own experiences, including the rape. Des had this uncanny ability, something we shared in common, that once she shined a light on her darkest moments, she could convert them into a tool to help her own growth as well as others. It is one of the many things that made us an outstanding team. She had walked in the victims' shoes and could provide the kind of empathy that only someone who had experienced trauma could provide. So many had had similar experiences: nearly 70 per cent of rape victims are assaulted by someone they know, and nearly half of them never report it or talk about it because they are ashamed, afraid of reprisals, or a combination of both. The work she did with the Help Line turned out to be very therapeutic, helping her cleanse the demons that had plagued her for such a long time. It also helped her develop a heightened understanding of patients' needs and make important use of her strong gift of empathy, which would later be so important in her work as a palliative care physician. Her ability to turn negatives into positives was astonishing.

"You know, Robert, she said one night after a long session at Help Line, "the reason this works so well is because I'm listening - truly listening - and that is the key to patient care. I wish more doctors understood this. These people are depressed, and that's a real sickness, to be sure, but think about all the critically ill people...people with serious and life-threatening illnesses. They really need someone to listen to them and be recognized as more than their illness. I know I will listen to my patients when I'm practicing medicine and encourage my colleagues to do the same. Many doctors don't realize how important it is!"

She had discovered something that often eludes people in the medical profession and, as the years would go by, that discovery would inform her interactions with every patient she touched, and every student she taught. Even then, her sensibilities were clearly in tune with palliative care discipline she would later go on to embrace and pioneer.

"It feels so good to be able to help others this way," she said many times. "And it's amazing how it actually helps me understand myself better! Guess I'm not the only one with demons."

I knew she must have heard some pretty rough stories and I was curious to know about them, but as much as I tried to get her to tell me some of the awful scenarios she tackled, she wouldn't. Those things were told to her in confidence, she said, and it would stay that way as far as she was concerned.

Things with us were good. We were both happy with our routine. I was the breadwinner - and still the family cook. Des tried her hand in the kitchen yet again, but it was always a disaster. She either under-cooked stuff or burned the hell out of it.

I actually enjoyed doing the cooking, even though I was working my ass off also, because in some sense, the cooking was more meaningful to me. The job never meant that much to me. I was never really into it. I was motivated purely by the money. I couldn't make it fast enough, because we sure knew how to spend it, so when I got a job offer for more money to be an Account Supervisor at a large financial PR and Investor Relations firm, I took it.

By now, Des had completed the first two years of medical school and was working on her PhD at CUNY/Mount Sinai, with plans to finish med school after. She was working with her advisor on a project that involved chicken eyes - the role of neuropeptides in altering synaptic receptors in the eyes of embryo chicks. This work had possible important scientific ramifications because these neuropeptides are pervasive in the brain and they are poised to affect synapses throughout the system.

Never much thought chick eyes were in any way like ours, but apparently, they are. This stuff was way too complicated for me to absorb, but I did my best to really understand it all because, although she seemed to be conquering her insecurities somewhat, there was still times that Des desperately needed affirmation of her abilities. I was the source of all love, acceptance, and praise, as well as the maker of some damned good rigatoni.

We were doing well and feeling great, and although I never went to the doctor myself, as far as I was concerned that didn't extend to Des. I knew from my mom and a close female cousin how important regular gynecological check-ups were, and I pressed Des to make an appointment. She resisted.

"I'm young and healthy!" she protested. "And besides, I'm too busy."

"Well, you don't take good enough care of yourself. I need you to be around for a long time!" I said.

"Not to worry, Robert," she laughed. "I'll be around for a long, long time. I didn't log in all this time with you for nothing."

"Come on," I said. "Do it for me. It'll be one of my birthday presents."

I gave her my best pleading look and smiled back. "I know," she said, about to repeat the line from one of her favorite movies that we had adopted as kind of an anthem. "Like Tom Cruise said in 'Jerry McGuire,'- 'You complete me.'"

It might have been a bit corny, but we really did feel that way and so, she finally agreed. One morning, a week later, I went with her for a check-up.

I remember teasing her. "Not sure I like that guy touching my stuff!"

She laughed and said, "Not to worry. The exam is anything but sexy."

I wanted to go into the exam room with her, but they wouldn't let me. The pregnant women in the waiting room all got a good laugh out of that one.

After what seemed like forever, Des finally came out into the waiting room. The doctor followed closely behind her, and I heard him say, "So, Desiree, it's nothing at all to worry about."

He gave her a big smile and nodded at me.

"See you back in a year for your regular check-up."

Des kinda smiled back at him.

"What did he mean 'nothing to worry about?'" I asked.

"Oh, nothing," Des said as we walked toward the reception desk.

The woman behind the desk handed her the bill and she passed it to me. "My banker will take care of it."

"Oh, that's so cute!" the receptionist said. She shot us a big smile.

I smiled back, but I was kind of anxious to get out of there and find out what the doctor meant by 'nothing at all to worry about.'

Des started for the door and I followed. The minute we were in the hallway, I asked.

"Oh, it was nothing, really," she answered. "He found a small lump, but he said it was consistent with dense, cystic breasts. I've had that forever. All the women in my family have cystic breasts."

I didn't like the word "lump," or the information about cystic breasts, for that matter, but this guy was a top-notch doctor and would never put his patients in harm's way.

"Don't worry," she said. "I trust him. He knows his stuff."

She gave me a big smile and tugged on my sleeve.

"Come on - it's a perfect day out there. Let's have lunch and be wicked for the rest of the day." She rubbed against me.

"Well, you're on for lunch," I said, "but I do have to get back to the office. Somebody's gotta fund this operation."

"You'll regret that remark when I'm a famous doctor and you're still writing financial press releases!" she jabbed.

Well, even though I was doing a hell of a lot more than writing financial press releases, I wasn't too thrilled with my job. Nonetheless, I really did have to get back to the office, but there was always time for a quick lunch and a short walk in the sunshine.

A few days after that, a headhunter contacted me about a position at a big firm as Senior Equity Analyst and Portfolio Manager for U.S. Technology and Telecommunications. The pay was good and the perks were great - an amazing 65 days of vacation, for starters. It sounded really good, but there was a catch - and a big one. I had to discuss it with Des.

I met her that evening at Jimmy's - our neighborhood haunt and the scene of our infamous reconciliation a few months before. It was crowded and noisy, but we managed two stools at the bar.

I told Des about the job.

"Wow! That sounds terrific!" she said. "What a great opportunity!"

Then I told her about the catch.

"Excuse me...the job is WHERE?" she asked, eyes as big as giant blue marbles.

"Abu Dhabi," I said.

"Abu what?"

"Dhabi," I laughed. "Abu Dhabi. As in The Emirates."

"The Emirates. Right. And can you tell me where the hell that is?"

I laughed again. My brilliant wife didn't know where The Emirates was.

"The United Arab Emirates."

"As in the middle of the desert?"

"Yes, but now they've got so much oil money, they've shoveled away a lot of the sand and are building fantastic new skyscrapers."

"Great," Des said. "The camels must really like that."

"Oh, they don't drive camels much anymore," I said. "More like Maserati's. They're really into expensive cars over there."

The curious look on her face faded.

"Well, it all sounds really interesting, but it's awfully far away Robert."

"I couldn't agree more," I said, actually relieved. While it would be an excellent career move, we were doing so well together, and had kind of hit our stride. At that point, the opportunity notwithstanding, I didn't really want to be that far away. As it was, Des would be moving to Toledo to finish up her PhD. The distance between New York and Toledo was only 500 miles. Hopping on a plane to spend weekends with Des would be easy. If I were in Abu Dhabi, it would have been a completely different scenario - a distance of more than 7000 miles, not to mention the time change which would complicate short visits. As far as I was concerned, I would pass.

So the next day, with Des hugging me from behind, I called the headhunter and said I wasn't interested. Just as soon as I got that out of my mouth, Des whispered, "But Robert, wait, just think of the fun we could have. We both love to travel and experience different cultures and we've never been in that part of the world." That was certainly true. We were always going off to someplace whenever we could get the chance. Then, almost as though he had overheard our conversation, the headhunter sweetened the pie: his client would fly both my wife and me, first class all the way, just to have a look.

"Robert - what fun!" Des said. "Let's go and at least have a look."

Des was so excited about the prospect of going that I figured what the hell. And so we went. We had a luxurious flight over, stayed in a five-star hotel, sunned ourselves at a beach club on the Persian Gulf, while being served fruity cocktails, took a boat ride in the incredible turquoise water, shopped in the timeless gold souk and ate delicious local cuisine, like Al Harees, kind of a meat stew that's slow-cooked with all kinds of exotic spices. I took tons of photos, of course, and we had a blast, and Des fell in love with the place.

When they made me a firm offer, Des was all over me to accept it.

"I love it here!" she said, as we were walking on the beach along the gulf. "You've just got to accept their offer, Robert. It will help us get out of debt."

That was certainly true.

"And I can come and visit every month, or we could meet in some romantic country in the middle." She paused, and then said quite earnestly, "You know you're not going to enjoy coming to Toledo."

That was certainly true, as well.

But she had that gleam in her eye. "We could travel..." Then she pressed up against me in that special way where I knew she would get her way. "...Europe, Morocco or even South Africa..."

It was certainly tempting. On top of the excellent pay and the beyond generous vacation days, they would be covering all my living expenses so, as Des had pointed out, it would give us a chance to get out of the hole. Of course, at that moment, I don't think either of us had taken into account what we would be spending for all the traveling.

"We have become so strong together," Des said, "we can handle the time apart, Robert, and this would be an amazing opportunity for you! You are so smart and good at what you do. This job will let you shine and open so many doors going forward. You could climb so high! Please don't pass it up. Let's think of your path, not just mine. And anyway, I will be in Toledo, Toledo, it certainly isn't a resort on the Persian Gulf."

What she said certainly made sense.

Then she asked with a huge smile and big blues sparkling with anticipation, "When else are we going to get the chance to do all that traveling. When we're 65?"

We both laughed at that...

While Des was totally convinced that my taking the job was a really good thing to do, I still had serious reservations. It was a long, long way from home and not exactly a place I had ever even thought about visiting, let alone living and working in without my wife. But in the end, at Des's urging, I made the commitment and signed the contract, which put me on board with the Abu Dhabi Investment Authority for two years.

But when it was time for me to go, Des was not upbeat. We were in the KLM boarding area at JFK, looking out at the huge, gleaming plane as it was being serviced and readied for flight. The seating area was crowded with businessmen, and there were a few families, with the women dressed in traditional Middle Eastern clothing, including varying degrees of facial cover.

"I don't know," Des said, hanging on to me. "It really *seemed* like a good idea..." Her usual big smile was absent.

"It *is* a good idea, Des," I re-iterated, all smiles on my end. "We can pay off our bills. "And like you said, we'd have all that travel that we both love!"

She had convinced me it was the right move to make, and now I was trying to convince her of the very same thing. And then the first boarding call came and Des's whole body went stiff. She squeezed my arm like a tourniquet.

"I'm going to hate this," she said. "Please don't go!" "And then the tears started to roll down her face.

Gee-sus...

"I know it's good for your career, and I want you to go, but I'm going to miss you so much..."

Then the tears turned into sobs.

I put my arms around her. "Baby, I have to go. You know I signed a contract." It would have been pretty messy to do an about turn at that point.

I lifted her chin. "We agreed - remember? Money...pay off our debts...travel..."

There was another boarding call and passengers were filing through the gate and onto the plane.

"You're going because you don't want to be with me anymore."

Dear God...Where did that come from?

"You're tired of me..."

With the exception of a few stragglers, by now just about everyone in the area had already boarded.

"Mr. Pardi. Last call. Mr. Robert Pardi, please board now."

That made Des cry even more. I felt helpless. I had to get on that plane.

"I've really got to go, Baby. How could I ever get tired of you? You are my life Baby and as you said, we are so strong now. We will make this work, I promise." I whispered.

She looked at me with so much pain on her face. I pulled her hands away from my arms. I felt like a murderer.

"This better not be the beginning of the end," she said.

I found myself laughing. Maybe it was a nervous reaction.

"Come on...you know that's hardly the case."

I headed for the gate, pulling Des by the hand. I could see the KLM attendant lean into the microphone.

"Mr. Robert Par..."

"I'm here...I'm here." I called over to her, but even as I answered, I then started asking myself, "is this what I really want to do?"

"Well, you had better hurry," the gate attendant said. "We're just about to close the gate."

I gave Des a hug, kissed her quickly on the forehead and dashed to the gate. The attendant checked my passport and boarding pass, and I was ushered forward. I was hard-pressed to move on - but I did. I turned around to see Des standing there all alone, a tissue in her hand. "I love you!" I yelled out. "Remember that I love you."

"And you know I love you," she called back. Her words rang in my ears and found myself asking myself over and over "should I really be getting on this plane?" as I walked through the passageway to the aircraft.

But I did get on the plane and the next eight hours were Hell. For the first couple of hours, I just sat in my First-Class seat, clutching a photo of Des, drinking all the free champagne they would give me while staring out the window. Then I made the mistake of watching a movie - "Jerry McGuire," of all things, and when they got to the part where he says, "you complete me," I nearly lost it. Why the Hell had I made such a stupid decision? There were lots of good jobs in the States.

I had a miserable layover in Amsterdam. The six hours seemed like six days and I didn't think the trip would ever be over. But my flight to Abu Dhabi was finally called and I settled into my seat for the last seven-hour leg of the trip.

I hadn't eaten for hours, but I didn't touch the food that had been placed in front of me. I remember the stewardess coming over to me right after the captain announced that we had begun the descent into the Abu Dhabi airport.

"Did you not care for the lunch, sir?" she asked.

I was kind of in a daze. She repeated her question. Then she said,

"You did not eat any of the food we served. Was it not to your liking?"

"Oh, no. Nothing like that."

"I can leave the tray with you for a few more minutes if you like."

"Thank you. But that's OK. I seem to have lost my appetite."

Then she gave me a big smile.

"Oh, you will get it back in Abu Dhabi, I am quite certain. You will love it there."

I remember that at that moment, the land mass came into view and loving it there was just about the last thing I thought could ever be possible.

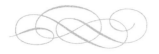

Chapter 11

The limo drive into Abu Dhabi from the airport seemed endless. Miles and miles of dusty road flanked by not much of anything. As we approached the city, the low-rise, muddy brown, tired-looking buildings that came into view didn't look as fun and interesting as they had when Des and I had seen them together. What seemed, then, to have a unique kind of charm to my westerner's eye now had no charm whatsoever. What the hell had I been thinking? My old job hadn't been that bad after all.

We entered the city and the newer, tall buildings that all the oil money had built came into view, but many of the streets were still small and narrow and we soon pulled into what was little more than an alleyway. We parked in front of the Hilton Residence Hotel, which, at that point, was the tallest building in Abu Dhabi.

"We're here, sir," the Indian driver said, looking at me through the rear-view mirror.

Great, I thought. *Home sweet fucking home.*

That was the first week of May,1997. I settled into what was really an amazing hotel apartment, with a full living room, two bedrooms and pretty decent furniture. I had a full view of The Gulf, and there was a nicely equipped gym, a large, top-floor pool and the staff couldn't have been nicer. Most of them were Indian and I soon learned that the bulk of workers in the Emirates was made up of Indians happy to find work in a growing economy.

I missed Des from the get-go, but if things worked out the way we had planned, we would visit each other every six weeks - when we weren't meeting in some wonderful place, that is. We had a big list of places we wanted to go: London, Amsterdam, Brussels, Luxembourg, Paris, Florence and Rome, for starters. She was already planning to come visit me in July, during her break from school, and I definitely was going to take her someplace special for her birthday in October. We were so looking forward to time together.

The second week I was there, my Grandmother Mary passed away, and as much as I adored her - my love, my champion, my role-model, the one person I could always turn to and who returned my love with every fiber of her body. I was not able to go to her funeral. My ironclad contract prohibited me from leaving Abu Dhabi for 30 days. I couldn't believe the timing. While I was devasted, I had said goodbye before I left, knowing it would be the last time I would ever see her. She had been very ill in the hospital and while she had stopped making sense when she spoke and didn't know most people when they came to visit, that day she reached out, grabbed me by the arm and said, "Robbie I love you."

"I love you too, Gram," I said and kissed her on the forehead.

That day is locked in my heart, as are so many of our days together. I used to call her Grandma Fella because she always said I was her fella. She never re-married after my grandfather - my father's father - died before I was born. One of the many reasons I loved her so much was that she was so different from my father. I never understood how he became such a miserable alcoholic with a mother like Grandma Fella. She was always so positive and so go-for-it in everything she did. She never learned to drive but that didn't stop her. She would just jump on a train and go wherever she liked with no fear whatsoever. She taught me to do that as well, she would tell me over and over to "live like a gypsy", to reach out beyond fear and live life. I knew that she would want me to embrace any path that would make me happy.

Des went to the funeral in my place and she called me right after to tell me about it. Everyone was surprised that I wasn't there, and Des had to defend me. My father, she reported, sniped "Yeah. He couldn't get a normal job in New York, like everybody else."

Apparently, he said it loudly enough so that even my grandmother could hear.

According to Des, my mother rushed to my defense. "Bob, he's sick about it," she said. "He adored his Nonna and you know it."

Even in front of my poor, dead grandmother, my father couldn't resist the chance to take a shot at me.

And although I was sad, I had to laugh thinking about Des in that sea of little old Italian ladies dressed in black, wringing their hands. Don't know how I would have handled it if the situation had been reversed and it had been me going to an Irish funeral.

Our lives went on. Des moved to Ohio, continued at school, and completed the first year of her PhD program, while I plunged into my Abu Dhabi Investment Authority Pension Plan job, analyzing US public stocks in the technical and telecom fields and then making strategic investments. It was challenging and when I wasn't concentrating on missing Des, I really got into it and made some pretty effective calls. It felt good to be on this strong career trajectory.

It came as a surprise to both of us, but it turned out that Des actually liked Ohio. The garden apartment near campus was modest, but she liked the area. It was rustic and so much more spacious than the cramped buildings on New York's upper east side where we had lived. What she liked most of all were the trees.

"I can't believe how much I love them, Robert!" she said. "There are trees everywhere I look. It's wonderful – and makes me feel good!"

Aside from being closer to nature, making new friends was also making her feel good. It was an experience that had really eluded her much of her life. She especially liked an Ethiopian woman named Adira, who was in the same PhD program. They had lots to talk about because Adira, also, was distanced from her husband, who remained back east in New Jersey where he was a Residence Director at a state school. Des and Adira spent many Friday nights together commiserating over beer and pizza.

But it was the neuropeptides embryo chick eyes experiment Des was working on that really got her juices going. She spent hours in that lab at her "rig," a large microscope tented over with nylon parachute fabric that was flanked by computers and other technical devices.

I had a difficult time picturing her there but when she sent me a photo, it was exactly as she described. Sometimes it was hard to relate to the fact that my wife was such a major brain. When you live with someone and share all that there is in a committed relationship, it's hard to fully understand that the person you sleep with every night and have stupid fights with and suffer through family events with is someone on their own, out of that context - and someone with such outstanding credentials having nothing to do with who you are as a couple. The same woman who tried to cook and failed so abysmally - but looked so cute doing it - and the same woman who could get me going at a moment's notice - was so brilliant. Even before publication of her PhD thesis, she co-authored an important paper in the 1995 issue of "Molecular Pharmacology" - *"P.C.P Type 1 Receptors Mediate Cyclic MP-Dependent Enhancement of Neuronal Acetylcholine Sensitivity."*

No, I didn't, and still don't, have a clue.

Yet with all of her achievements, and all the work she had done on herself, Des was still plagued with self-doubts. Like her weight. She was constantly obsessing about it, which was ridiculous. She was hardly overweight. She rarely missed a day at the gym and worked as hard there as she did in the lab. Sometimes I blamed myself. I had always been a gym rat, and when I initially got her going to a health club near our New York apartment, I never thought it would turn into an obsession.

Whatever we both were doing, once a week, we always made time for a phone call. Between the eight-hour time difference and our work commitments, the calls were sometimes hard to schedule, but we always made it work.

And then there were the impromptu calls, like one day when I was in an important meeting. There I was, seated around a conference table with a bunch of suits...well, actually *dishdashas*, the common name for the traditional white *kanduras* that Emirati men wear. I was addressing the group about an investment opportunity I thought was especially interesting when my secretary, a young Indian man, knocked on the door, opened the door a crack, and ventured his head in.

"Mr. Pardi, so sorry to interrupt," he whispered, "but you have a call on line 1."

I was really annoyed because I had specifically said that I did not want to be interrupted.

"I told you, Baliji - no calls."

"But it's your wife, Mr. Pardi," Baliji said. "She says it's important."

Leaving a room filled with middle eastern men to take a call from your wife was not exactly the way to win friends and influence people in that part of the male-dominated world, but I was concerned. Was something wrong? Was she sick?

I excused myself and left the room. I picked up the phone at Baliji's desk.

"Des...what is it? Are you all right?"

There was a giggle at the other end of the line.

"Oh, I'm fine. And you would be so proud of me! I'm making a meatloaf."

She called me out of a meeting to tell me she was doing what?

"It's just that I can't find the aluminum foil."

Can't find the what?!

I couldn't believe the conversation.

"I'm cooking a meat loaf," she said, "and I can't find the aluminum foil. I have to cover it, don't I?"

I had to laugh. It was too ridiculous and just so Desiree.

"You do know that you got me out of an important meeting with some real heavy hitters so you could ask me about aluminum foil?" I laughed some more...we both laughed.

"Oh, I'm sorry, Robert. But it's important. I'm cooking! When you come back home, I'm going to cook for you - every night!"

Right. While attending med school classes and doing rounds at the hospital and researching intern slots and studying for the boards...

In her mind, I guess it was important because she sure as hell couldn't cook and that fact that she was trying, in the midst of her chick embryo experiments and paper writing and God knows what else, it was good enough for me. And I knew she missed the ordinary moments that we used to share together, because I sure missed them too. And even though it had been a beyond inconvenient interruption, I was happy to hear her voice.

I went back into that meeting wearing a big smile, which my colleagues couldn't figure out because whatever had been important enough to get me out of that meeting in the first place surely had to have been urgent. I must have looked like an idiot because I couldn't stop grinning. Even 7,000 miles away, that girl could put a smile on my face.

In addition to our weekly phone calls, there were letters just about every day. This was in 1997, and we didn't have personal email yet, so we wrote letters to each other in long hand. I'd never been a serviceman stationed an ocean away from home, but that's what it must have felt like getting a letter from your girl.

Des's letters were chatty - mundane stuff, like the nightly pillow talk we both missed so much...the kinds of things that keep couples close. Des wrote on lined, three-ring paper, like a schoolgirl.

"Remember on 'Sabrina,' the boyfriend was supposed to find out that she was a witch? Well..."

Hard to believe, but my brainiac wife was addicted to sit-coms.

"I bought two low-fat cookbooks today. I am trying a recipe tomorrow for grilled chicken. You cut all of the fat off first..."

That fat obsession - both on her body and in her food.

"I'm going to sleep now because I have cycling class first thing in the morning. I've got to keep my weight down."

More weight obsession. It didn't occur to either of us at the time, but she was probably anorexic - triggered, most likely, by the stress of finishing her PhD, our being apart and, as we later learned, of seriously low self-esteem.

Sometimes she would make bizarre observations about things that no one else would go near.

"Did I ever tell you that I noticed people put their fingers in their ears to get out the ear wax - and then they eat it?"

Only Desiree would comment on something like that. She could be really funny. But there were plenty of not-so-fun letters, too - the letters that made me hate myself for following the money.

"This was such a mistake," she wrote. "Why are we doing this? It's like we are separated. Are we separated? Have you fallen out of love with me?"

Of course not...

"I could never imagine my life without you. You mean the world to me, Robert. You know that, don't you?

I did know that, and she certainly meant the world to me.

Sometimes the letters were very dark.

"I had this dream about the apocalypse. It was awful. All the fire and the destruction and dead people everywhere. It happened here, but you were over there without me and you survived. You were finally free."

Free? That was the last thing in the world I wanted to be. There were many letters like that and they tore at my heart, and the only thing I could do was to reassure her by phone, by letter and during our frequent meetings that we were as solid as ever.

The great trips we were able to take helped to get us through. Des was really into travel and she loved researching fun places for us to go. One of the best times we ever had was on a European train, kind of like the Orient Express that was immortalized by Agatha Christie. We put our own spin on Inspector Poirot and Miss Marple, starting off in Paris, then closing ourselves off in our private cabin as we moved on to Lausanne, Milan and finally Venice. The days and nights we spent on that trip left us feeling totally secure about our marriage and the choices we had made. We were young, we were in love, and we were both on paths leading to big careers. We were the lucky ones.

I especially remember a late lunch in the dining car as we were going through the magnificent Italian countryside, covered with fields of yellow *girasoles*, huge sunflowers bending up to the sun-filled sky.

Des was glowing. "This has been such a great trip!" she said. "Now I'm really ready to plunge back in and finish up my PhD." A glorious smile lit up her face. "And then, maybe we can do this again before I go back for my last two years of med school!"

"Sure," I laughed. "Just give me some time to rob the Emirates Treasury."

"But Snoopy," she said, "what are we going to do? Wait until we're 65?"

"You're right," I agreed, as I got up to hit the loo. I leaned down and kissed her on the forehead. "That'll never be us!"

Des smiled up at me. "Never..."

When I returned and approached the table, I couldn't help but to stop and just look at her. She was facing the window, enjoying the sun on her face. I will always remember how peaceful and happy she looked that day. She was the picture of contentment.

A few days later Des went back to Ohio and I returned to Abu Dhabi and the glow of the wonderful holiday soon faded. And it wasn't just Des who had mood swings. I frequently found myself worrying about her being out there alone, and the men who might be hitting on her. She was beautiful, had the kind of body that drove men nuts - and she was alone without me to protect her. My imagination went wild. I even started to worry that while she was out with her girlfriends, some guy might slip something in her drink. Many nights I consoled myself with too much to drink, which was not a good thing. Despite having wanted to be different from my father, I seemed to have too much of a liking for the stuff. I was afraid I'd follow in his footsteps. But that fear didn't seem to stop me. I'd sit in my dark apartment and down one too many scotches one too many times - when I wasn't out drinking with the boys, that is. Don't believe what you hear about there being no alcohol in the middle east, by the way. If that were the case, there'd be no westerners pulling down big bucks at big jobs.

What the fuck had I gotten myself into? I missed Des terribly, and with all our trips, we were spending it faster than I could make it. It was starting to make no sense - no sense at all - and I seriously considered trying to get out of my contract. But Des was working so hard in school and loved the traveling so much, there was no way that I could deprive her of it. The pressure she felt, albeit possibly self-imposed, was intense, and the reprieves that the travel afforded were good. I wanted her to have the excitement and I started to think I could make the best decisions for her. So, of course, we planned another trip - this time to Spain and Morocco for Christmas.

We were sitting under a large umbrella, sipping drinks, at the pool at our hotel in Tangiers. Des seemed really content, so she surprised me when she said, "These vacations are amazing - and I love you for working your ass off to afford this for us - but the only time I'm really happy is when I'm with you. I'm absolutely miserable when I get home."

I knew exactly how she felt. "Baby, you know it's the same for me."

"No, it can't be," she said. "It's different for a woman. Sometimes I'm ready to pack in the whole med school thing and just be a housewife."

A housewife! You could have knocked me down with the proverbial feather. She had never wanted to be a housewife and was ambivalent, at best, about having kids, although in the years that followed, she loved being an aunt to her sister's child and to my brother's daughter.

"I'm not sure I'd make the best mother," she said more than once. "And aside from the fact I've always wanted to be a doctor - and a really good one - I love what we have together, just the two of us, and I never want that to change. But it's not right," she said, looking at me pleadingly. "Why should I have to choose between my husband and my career?"

Women were already starting to have it all, so this came as a surprise - and especially since she was such an academic over-achiever.

"I love what we have together, and I'm thinking that my decision to get both an MD and a PhD is stopping us from sharing so much together. I love you so much and want so much to give you everything I have and make you happy."

"Baby, I know that," I said. "And you do make me happy. I am so, so proud of you. And you don't have to choose, Des. You're going to have both. You do have both. This arrangement is just temporary."

Even as I said it, I realized that temporary was turning into a very long time. But no way was I going to encourage her to let go of her dream. She had worked way too hard. And she had what it takes to be one hell of a doctor – the knowledge, the drive and, as we later learned when she became a palliative care pioneer, the crucial empathy that could make all the difference in the lives of patients and their families.

"In the scheme of things, you don't have that much longer to go. Keep your eye on the ball."

Des did not seem in any way convinced, but I really wasn't ready to talk about it anymore - not without carefully thinking it through in all of its ramifications.

"Come on," I said. "It's a gorgeous day. Let's soak it all up while we have the chance."

Des pouted for a bit, then smiled and all was good again. She went back of course, did her thing and the following October, got her PhD.

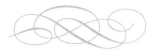

Chapter 12

O ur ninth wedding anniversary coincided with Des's receiving her PhD. A big celebration was in order, so of course I would fly home. We always managed to be together for anything major, and certainly for birthdays and anniversaries. I planned a dinner at a great Italian restaurant in the neighborhood with family and friends, including Dave, my closest friend and his partner Daryl, and Adira, her Ohio friend and her husband. I wanted to go all out and take everyone to a fancy place, but Des said she preferred one of our familiar haunts to just an impersonal, high-tech, mid-town space.

Like a bunch of rambunctious kids on prom night, we all piled into a huge white stretch limo and drove around town taking turns hooting out of the opening in the roof. Even Des's mom and my father stuck their heads out, which made us all smile. Everyone was in good spirits and we took over a corner of the restaurant and had enough to eat and drink to feed an army: *bruschetta*, fried *calamari*, a choice of pastas, some great *ossobucco*, *bronzino* and some perfect *broccoli di rabe* sauted with garlic...and lots of red wine, of course. Everyone seemed relaxed and to be enjoying themselves. Des's parents were beaming with pride, and that made Des feel great.

Just before dessert, I offered a toast to Des.

"So, everyone, please lift your glass and join me in congratulating my wife, Desiree Ann Pardi, PhD - the most amazing woman you will ever meet. There's nothing she can't do when she puts her mind to it!"

"*Salute!*" and "Here, here!" came from around the table.

Des popped up from her chair. "I need to thank my wonderful husband for all of his support. I could never have done this without him," she said to everyone. Then she turned to me. "And thank you, Robert, for nine wonderful years together. Happy anniversary!"

"Happy anniversary!" I wished her back as I put my arms around her and kissed her.

There were more toasts, all around, from our friends and parents and it was really a nice evening, but we were both anxious just to get home and be alone for our very own celebration. So after quick good-byes, we left and went back to our old east-side apartment for one of the last times. We had kept it for our visits to New York, but would soon be letting it go because Des had decided to take a year off to live with me in Abu Dhabi before returning to med school. I was happy that she had made that decision and we were both looking forward to much needed, extended time together.

But before going to Abu Dhabi, we planned to celebrate Des's 31st birthday in one of her favorite places. So, a couple of days later, we packed up, took Dollar$ to my parents, and flew to Paris. I had sprung for first class on Air France and it was worth every penny. It was luxurious and the flight attendants kept the *Veuve Cliquot* coming. Des was coming down the home stretch with her schooling - although there were still years of med school, interning, residency and fellowships ahead - and I was pulling in the bucks in my job. Best of all, we had beaten the odds of staying in love through so many ups and downs and months and months of separation. We were happy. We were chasing life.

Our room at the Bristol was picture perfect and we celebrated Des's birthday with a picnic lunch near Notre Dame, a long walk by the Seine and a wonderful dinner at a small, family-owned bistro. The husband and wife owners serenaded Des with "*Bon*

Anniversaire" and she just loved it, beaming up at them with her beautiful smile. It was a wonderful night, made all the more perfect because we knew we were about to have a whole year together.

After a few more days of walks around the city, incredible meals, some marathon shopping - and, of course, some quality room time - we were back on Air France, this time headed for Abu Dhabi.

An hour into the six-hour trip, we were both settled comfortably in our seats, reading. I was catching up on a couple of days' worth of the *Wall Street Journal* and Des was into her latest bodice-ripper. I never understood how a woman with such intellectual and academic chops liked those books, but she sure did! Guess they were a fun break from the seriousness of the scientific stuff that filled her long days.

"So, has he seduced her yet?" I chided.

But instead of her usual quip and smile, Des turned to me with a pained expression on her face.

"What's wrong?" I put my hand on her arm.

She eased her arm away.

"What's wrong?" I asked again.

"Oh, nothing. Just a pain under my arm. It'll go away." She squirmed a bit, then went back to her book.

Probably nothing, like she said, I thought, as I dozed off.

When I awoke, the cabin lights were dimmed. Most of the passengers were sleeping, but I was surprised to see that Des was not in her seat. I got up, looked in the refreshment area in the front and checked the first-class bathrooms. No sign of her.

I spotted the flight attendant and asked if she had seen my wife.

"*Ah, oui.*" she responded. "She is walking down at the other end of the plane. Apparently she could not sleep."

At that moment, I saw Des approaching.

"Anything wrong, sweetie?" I asked.

"Can't sleep," she said. "Maybe I shouldn't have had that fancy dessert."

"Ah, but you deserved it," I said. "Come on. Let's go back to our seats."

We walked through the darkened cabin and settled back in, but in a few moments, Des turned to me. "Actually, I'm a little worried about this pain under my arm. Remember that lump doctor Grant said was nothing? Well, the pain is on the same side."

Fear shot through my body. "Oh, I'm sure that's just a coincidence. You probably pulled something when we were dealing with the luggage." I said it with a smile, but...

"Don't think so," Des said, shaking her head. "I can feel the lump, now. It must have gotten bigger because I couldn't feel it before." She took my hand and placed it next to her breast. I pressed in with my fingers and froze. I could feel it. I could also feel the blood drain from my body.

Stay positive, I said to myself. *Just stay positive.* "It's probably a cyst," I said, "like you've had before. We'll get you checked out as soon as we get to Abu Dhabi. You need a physical to get your residency papers anyway."

I put my arm around her. "Don't worry, honey," I said in the most soothing voice I could muster, hoping the fear hadn't broken through the forced smile on my face, because it sure had landed in the bottom of my stomach.

The next day we went to the hospital in Abu Dhabi. I stood by in the room as the doctor, a British-Jordanian from London, examined Des. He was pleasant, but on the serious side, and didn't say much. After he finished the exam, he and I walked out into the hall together.

"Mr. Pardi," the doctor said, clearing his throat, "Mrs. Pardi..."

"Dr. Pardi," I found myself correcting this doctor. "My wife has her PhD."

"Ah, yes," he said with a slight smile. "She did mention her background. Impressive". He cleared his throat again. "Dr. Pardi was quite right. There is a lump there. I don't think it is anything to be alarmed at, but to be on the safe side, we need to do a needle aspiration."

He may as well have been speaking Arabic.

"Needle aspiration? What, exactly, is that?"

"It's quite straight forward," the doctor replied. "Cells from the suspicious area are removed and sent to a laboratory for analysis to determine if there's any malignancy."

Malignancy. Fear clutched my body and threatened to double me over. *Cancer. This couldn't be possible. My wife couldn't have cancer. She's only 31 years old.*

"You need to go to The American Hospital in Dubai," the doctor continued, "and see my colleague, Dr. Al Abjani. He will take care of it."

I knew about the American hospital in Dubai from the ex-pat community. It had a great reputation. Knowing that, however, didn't help the terror that I felt.

The doctor smiled then patted me on the shoulder. "I will make the arrangements straight away."

I must have looked really upset because he came back with, "Do not worry. It is nothing. She will be fine."

Of course she will be. This whole thing is a mistake - a huge mistake.

At that point, I looked past the doctor and could see Des through the open door. She was sitting on the edge of the bed. She gave me her usual, up-beat, sweet smile.

The doctor started to walk away, and I stopped him.

"Doctor, won't you be going back in to tell her?" I asked.

"Oh, I think it will be better if you relay the information," he said. Then he nodded at me and continued walking away.

At first I thought his not telling Des directly might have been due to cultural differences in that male-centric part of the world, but I later learned that he was so stunned at suspecting cancer in such a young, vibrant woman, nearly a physician herself, that he felt more comfortable telling her husband.

"So the doctor says that just to be on the safe side, we have to do a needle aspiration."

"That's what I figured," Des said cheerfully. "No big deal."

We left the hospital and stopped for some Turkish coffee before heading back to the apartment. Des was very dismissive of the whole thing.

"It's nothing...I'm sure of it," she said, smiling.

I tried my best to match her positive mood, but I wondered if that's how she really felt. As for me, I felt like the world had begun to implode.

The next day we drove the 130 kilometers - 80 miles - to Dubai. It took about an hour and a half, and we bantered back and forth about nothing especially meaningful, trying to stay light and positive. We listened to music, a wonderful Lebanese singer named Inglesia, and Ricky Martin who was living his best *Vida Loca*.

The American Hospital in Dubai is staffed with US-trained doctors and it is state-of-the-art. We had both been relieved to learn that and when we saw the ultra-modern facility, we squeezed each other's hand.

"It'll all going to be OK." I said, "but we best not hold hands going in." It was important to be respectful of the local customs, which frowned on public displays of affection between men and women.

"I know it will be OK," Des responded cheerfully. "I'm only 31 - way too young for anything serious."

"Way too young," I echoed, trying hard to believe it as the words came out of my mouth.

So they did the needle aspiration, and once again the doctor spoke to me. This time he was an "Anglo-Egyptian with unexpected blue eyes and a British accent to match.

"There was no fluid in the aspirate," he said. "This is not good, Mr. Pardi. It predisposes to suspicious cells."

"Suspicious cells." My mind raced. "You mean cancerous?"

"Frankly, that's a strong possibility. We need to do a full biopsy and send it to our colleagues at The Mayo Clinic for analysis."

The Mayo Clinic... How I wished we were home on our own familiar turf. "How long will it take to get the results?" I asked.

"Not long," he answered. "A few days."

A few days! It sounded like an eternity.

But there was no choice, so they did the biopsy and Des handled it like a champ. "I'm impressed with how competent they are," she said cheerfully as we left the hospital later that day. "And nice. They're just being extra cautious, as they should be. It's probably nothing." Then she laughed. "It's really funny how they talk to you and not to me. But, you know what? I kinda like it. There's something comforting about having you as my buffer." She smiled and continued talking as though she had said nothing unusual. At that moment, of course, we had no way of knowing that my being Des's buffer would come to define our way of handling things in the future.

Des then gave me one of her mega-watt smiles and kissed me on the cheek. "How lucky am I that you are my husband!"

"Be careful," I joked, trying to stay light-hearted. "We don't want to get thrown in jail!"

"Oh, I keep forgetting," Des laughed. "Just as long as we can do what we want at home."

I winked at her. "I'll second that!" Des was so sure it was nothing. I wanted so much to be as sure as she was.

A few days later, the doctor called me at my office.

"Mr. Pardi, your wife's test came back," he said, and then he paused. "I am afraid the news is not very good."

"She has cancer," I whispered, not wanting to hear the words come out of my mouth, let alone his.

"Yes," he said, "and we recommend removal of the tumor as soon as possible."

I stopped breathing and my mind careened into a bottomless, black pit. *Cancer. Death. She's going to die.*

"Mr. Pardi, are you there?"

"Yes," I managed to answer. *My God. I can't...no I won't think that way...* "It's...it's...just we'll need some time to figure things out."

"Of course," he said. "But get back to me as soon as you can."

I hung up the phone and began to sob. I can't remember ever crying like that before, even when I learned my grandmother had died. How was I ever going to tell Des? I left the office and went home. I was devastated but had to keep myself as up as possible. I had to be strong. It was imperative.

Des was at the desk near the window. She loved to sit there because several parakeets had nested inside the crevices in the outside wall and one of them, a little yellow and green fellow she had named Abdul, liked to visit with her.

She looked up when she heard me come in.

"Abdul, looks who's home!" she said with a big smile.

I must have had an awful expression on my face because her smile quickly faded.

"There's something important I need to tell you."

"Not sure I want to hear it," she said, shaking the bird from her finger. Then she looked at me quite directly. "Did you get fired?"

How I had wished that's all it was. I shook my head then walked over and took her hand. "The doctor called a little while ago..."

She pulled her hand away then quickly said, "No. I absolutely don't want to hear it."

"Des, honey, you have to. The doctor called with the results of the biopsy." I took a deep breath. "Suspicious cells were found, and they want to do a lumpectomy as soon as possible."

Des looked at me for what seemed like forever and then shook her head. A procedure like that here, in Dubai," she said calmly.

"I don't think so." She thought for a moment. "The first thing I need to do is to talk to Dr. Palokas."

Dr. George Palokas, in New York, was Des's primary care doctor and she thought the world of him, so that was clearly the judicious thing to do. I totally agreed, and we spent several anxious hours before we could reach him. Once we did and had the test results faxed, he concurred with the local doctor: the lumpectomy needed to be done asap.

We wanted to go back home for the procedure, but it was the end of Ramadan and a few days before Thanksgiving, and as hard as we tried and as many calls as we made, we could not get flights back to the States.

"There is no time to waste, by the time you get back and we set everything up I fear it could be months given we are heading into the holiday season." Dr. Palokas advised. "Get it done in Dubai."

So our course was charted. We scheduled the lumpectomy for two days later - the first possible available time. The amazing thing about the Emirates was the speed at which things could get done as well as their having the latest medical equipment. When I walked into the recovery room after the procedure, I could hear the monitors humming and the IV apparatus clicking with that steady, metronome precision. Surgical tapes were visible from under Des's hospital gown, tubes protruded from under her arms and from her nostrils, and fluids were flowing into her veins.

I swallowed hard at the sight of her like that. *How could this possibly be happening? My brilliant, beautiful, healthy, young wife.* I sat down in the chair and waited for her to wake up. When she did, sometime later, she smiled weakly at me, but before I could say a word, she looked down at her arm and then followed the lead up to the IV drip.

"Oh, no!" she yelled. "No!"

I got up and put my hand on her shoulder. She tried to sit up but fell back on her pillow.

"It's bad, isn't it? I knew if I woke up with a morphine drip that it would be bad." Des looked at me hard. "It's stage 3, isn't it?"

"We don't know yet.

What the hell is stage three? I thought. I was not at all versed in the language of cancer.

She bolted up. "Don't tell me anything, Robert. Please. I don't want to know. I just want it off!"

"You can't take the IV off, sweetie. Your body need those fluids."

"Not the fluids, Robert. The breast. I want the damn breast off – and I want it off as fast as possible!"

I will never forget that look of sheer determination on her face. Nor will I forget how I felt when the doctors told me the extent of the cancer. I thought I would fold up right then and there and never stand up straight again. In a heartbeat life changed as did my vocabulary. They had removed 12 lymph nodes during the procedure and 11 were cancerous. The diagnosis: Stage 3B HER2 neu positive breast cancer, a particularly aggressive form of breast cancer that was hard to treat at that point in time. Today's newer drugs, such as Herceptin, were not yet available.

How could this possibly be? My wife was young, healthy, a newly minted PhD and halfway through medical school. The God that I had been brought up to trust and believe in couldn't have had this plan for her.

Desiree was adamant. She did not want the details, and I respected her wishes. When I thought about her decision not to know those specifics, it was not at all surprising. In school, she had never wanted to know her grades - only whether or not she had passed or failed - not that failing had even been a remote possibility. When grades were posted, it had been my job to look them up and report back to her. I had always wanted to scream "All A's, Sweetie. All A's," but always stuck to her wishes and simply told her that she had passed. The same had been true of the MCATs, the tests for medical school admission and later on for her medical board scores.

"Great! She would say with a big smile. "Now I can breathe." She had done her best and only wanted to know that she had passed. She didn't want to be judged, she often said. "I felt judged my whole life. Now I can live my life differently."

How I wished we were dealing with something as simple as her grades - but we weren't. Nonetheless, even without knowing the specifics, Des wanted the breast removed. No one questioned her decision - neither Dr. Palokas or the local doctor - and certainly not me.

"Robert, I feel so bad that you have to go through all of this with me. I know it will not be easy for you."

And I knew it wouldn't, but I would always be there for her. "You would do the same for me, Des. We will always be there for each other - a team right!"

"Yes we will," she said, squeezing my hand.

So we made the arrangements for the operation. We tried to stay positive and the doctor was so helpful in that regard. "This procedure will go a long way toward getting you healthy," he said, and Des chose to look at it that way.

"I just love this doctor's attitude. He's so empathetic," she said. "I can't imagine any surgeon at home having that level of patient understanding. He really listens to me and you know how important I think that is."

Like not wanting to know specifics and my acting as her buffer would define the way we dealt with Des's cancer, this way of thinking about a patient's needs would later characterize Des's approach to treating patients as whole human beings, and not focusing only on their disease - one of the foundations of palliative care.

What neither of us realized, at the time, was that this was the beginning of Des's palliative care consciousness. The palliative care movement, the recognition that in addition to receiving serious and effective pain management, patients have a right to put their personal goals front and center when embarking on a course of treatment for a serious disease such as cancer, was barely making a ripple at that time. This was to change dramatically in the ensuing few years and Des would go on to play an important role.

Des wanted to do something fun the night before the procedure and the doctor was all for it. "You absolutely should!" he said, and once again, we loved his attitude. He suggested a lovely spot near Dubai Creek where we could have dinner, and even recommended that Des have some wine. She could have picked anything in the world that she wanted to do or anyplace she wanted to go and I swear I would have made it happen, but Des liked that idea, so that's what we did.

We left the hospital and Des had drips taped to her leg and to the port that had been installed so that she could have continuous infusions of pain medication. It was cumbersome getting around, but Des wanted to go and so we would. I would have carried her on my back, had it been necessary.

The restaurant was charming and we sat at a candle-lit table overlooking the water. Even with all the tubes and drips, Des still looked so beautiful against the reflection of the water. It was hard to imagine that she had such a monster growing in her body.

And her attitude was extraordinary. I marveled at it.

"It's like the doctor said, Robert. This procedure will go a long way toward getting me healthy, and we should celebrate getting me healthy."

While I had to struggle to match her mood, I was determined to do it. I lifted my glass of wine. "To celebrating getting you healthy."

"To celebrate getting me healthy," she joined in.

As our glasses clicked, I so hoped that would be the outcome.

The next day, which was Thanksgiving Day, 1998, at the age of 31, my beautiful, brilliant, PhD and soon-to-be-physician wife had her right breast removed. She was in the hospital for four days and not once did she ask for any specifics about her condition. It was clear, by then, how we would be dealing with things going forward.

"My wife doesn't want to know any of the specifics," I told the doctor, "so please relay all the information to me."

Des may have wanted the breast to come off from the get-go, but as it turned out, the tumor margins were not clear so it would have had to come off anyway. It's called "reducing the tumor burden," the doctor said, as I plunged into the esoterica of a whole new language - the language of cancer that I ironically might have learned had I not made the decision years before to drop out of pre-med to chase the money.

There were moments in the hospital when fear gripped my whole body, but I vowed I would conquer it, and never let Des see that I entertained anything less than totally positive thoughts - but if I could have gotten a hold of that doctor in New York who, the year before, had told her that the lump they both felt was nothing, I would have torn the bastard's heart out.

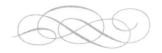

Chapter 13

It's true. Laughter really is the best medicine and as was typical Des, she filed our home with it. For the next two weeks, while Des was healing, we watched every cartoon we could find, and surprisingly, we found quite a few American favorites in one of the least American places in the world. We rooted for Tweety and cheered every time he outwitted Sylvester, roared every time Bugs Bunny chomped on a carrot or asked "What's Up Doc?' and doubled over when Elmer Fudd couldn't pronounce his R's and said "waabit" over and over again while he was running his perennially losing race to do in our boy Bugs.

Des was amazing, never once wanting to talk about cancer in a negative way or bemoan what she had facing her. When I would try to ease her into a conversation, she would just say that there would be plenty of time for that and it can't become the focal point of our lives.

I stayed home to look after her. No way was I going to the office. Work was the farthest thought from my mind. I changed her dressings, massaged her arm to prevent the lymphedema that so often accompanies lymph node removal, made sure she ate properly and was her constant cheerleader. When she was sleeping and I was not at her side, I researched breast cancer, specifically the kind of breast cancer Des had and the recommended courses of treatment.

Over and over again, she asked how I was doing and told me how grateful she was that I was there for her. Of course I was. She would have been there for me in a heartbeat. We were a team.

It was a strange cancer - not that all of them aren't strange - in that the cancerous cells were mostly in the tissue surrounding the breast and only in the very tip of the tumor itself. Google didn't exist then, but at least I had access to the internet and Yahoo and was able to find information. Research without the internet would have been virtually impossible, so I was thankful for that resource.

Even before we would go on to interview doctors, Des was very clear on how she wanted things to go and reiterated her decision: "I only want to know what I absolutely have to know to continue going forward," she said. "Not the number of lymph nodes involved, not the size of the tumor, the drugs I'm going to get or the dosages - and no survival stats or prognosis. I want only the most basic information.

I would be the receiver of all the information and the conduit to any and all the doctors. This was going to put enormous pressure on me and Des was so concerned about that.

"I worry that this is going to be too heavy of a burden for you, Robert. I really do." Her eyes were full of love when she said that on so many occasions and that only deepened my commitment.

It seemed like the logical way to do things, a natural progression, albeit years later, from the way things were when we were at Stony Brook together: no specific grades, only if she had passed or failed. And she only wanted information funneled through me.

So here I was checking her grades again, so to speak. "And, if that's what made the whole thing easier for her, it was fine with me, because more than anything, I needed to be part of her cure. What I didn't realize at the time, however, was the quantum shift our relationship had taken. From years of Des being subtly in control, the reins had been placed squarely in my hands.

Two weeks after the mastectomy, just before we left to go back to the States, Des and I took a walk along the Gulf. Des had always loved the beach and the sun, and the Gulf is a spectacular body of water with startling stripes of blue, green and aqua that glisten like huge jewels. I was happy that this heavenly stretch of sand and water was there for her.

"Cancer is not going to be the center of my life," she declared with a big smile, her face lifted to catch the sun's rays. "I have a lot to do, now more than ever, and I'm just going to live around it. I know I am asking a lot of you Robert and a lot is going to fall on you. I know you've said we are a team and that I've said this before, but I worry... I worry so about the burden on you. I only ever wanted to bring you happiness, joy and love. This may be too much. Are you with me?"

Was I with her? Burden? I would gladly have taken the cancer in her place. At that point, I really regretted not having gone to medical school. *Maybe if I had, I could cure her,* I thought.

"You know I'm with you, Baby. I'll do anything - absolutely anything. I'd swap places with you in a heartbeat if I could. It's us, together, forever and always."

"I know you would Robert and then it would be me wanting to swap places with you."

She squeezed my hand, as she so often did when words couldn't possibly tell the story. And I squeezed back. We stood for a long moment and looked out at the beauty of the sea on what, judging from the surroundings, should have been a perfect day.

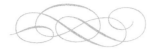

Chapter 14

As resolute as Des was that cancer would not be the center of her life, the cancer had to be dealt with, so she had to postpone her return to med school to finish her last two years. Her personal leave turned into a medical leave. What I was realizing was the cancer had to become the center of my life to allow her to live around it, and not become the center of our life. It had to center itself in me in order to protect her coping mechanisms.

The next day, a week after the mastectomy, we went back to New York to find the right oncologist. Khaled Al-Muhairy, a young Emirati with whom I worked at the Investment Authority and to whom I had grown close, insisted that we accept a gift of first-class tickets to New York on British Airways. It's considered an insult, in the Middle East, not to accept someone's gift, so we did. It would prove to be the first of many selfless acts of kindness on the part of this man with whom I would go on to form a very close business association and a relationship more akin to being brothers than just friends.

We arrived in New York, checked into a midtown hotel and started on the round of interviews that we had set up with the help of Dr. Palokas.

We'd heard about Evangeline Ladrin, a bright, young oncologist at an important hospital and decided that we should see her first. When I called her office to arrange for the appointment for the day after we arrived home, I made it very clear that Des did not wish to hear the specifics of her cancer at that or any other time going forward. The secretary hesitated for a moment, then said she would pass the information along to the doctor.

The morning we went to the appointment, Des was in good spirits. We arrived at Dr. Ladrin's office right on time and, after a brief wait, the secretary announced that the doctor was ready to see us.

"My husband needs a word with the doctor first," Des informed the secretary.

"But we..."

"I'll be just a minute," I said, pushing for what I felt were crucial minutes alone with the doctor.

The secretary was reluctant, but she nodded and ushered me into Dr. Ladrin's office. It was white and sterile and the doctor, an attractive but no-nonsense-looking, young woman, was sitting behind an uncluttered desk. I walked over and extended my hand.

"Well, clearly you are not Mrs. Pardi," she said, without so much as a smile.

Nonetheless, I smiled back. "Robert Pardi," I said. "Dr. Pardi's husband."

"Yes," she said, with a stiff shake.

"You're aware that my wife has her PhD and is halfway through medical school?" I asked. I thought it was important for the doctor to know Des's background.

I could see the impatience in her eyes.

"Yes, yes...go on."

"Well, it may seem unusual to you, Dr. Ladrin, but my wife does not want to know the specifics of her disease."

"Excuse me," she said, leaning forward.

"I informed your secretary when I made the appointment."

She paused. "She did mention something like that," Dr. Ladrin said, "but it's totally irregular."

I took that in before answering.

"I was very clear with your assistant," I said. I felt frustration creeping out of all of my pores and I struggled to control it. "At any rate," I said calmly, "we're discussing it now."

I could feel her impatience graduating to annoyance.

"My wife made the decision when this whole thing started that in order for her to cope with her situation and pursue her goals, she would prefer not to hear the details of her breast cancer and to have all of the information funneled through me." I paused for a moment and looked her directly in the eye. "I know the extent of what she will be able to handle."

I will always remember the look the doctor gave me in return. It was somewhere between incredulity and disbelief, with a whole lot of contempt thrown in for good measure.

"The patient, herself, needs to be informed," she fired back.

We stared hard at one another, the tension broken only when her secretary knocked and opened the door.

"We're running behind, Doctor," she said.

Dr. Ladrin disengaged from me and turned to her secretary.

"Yes. Please show Dr. Pardi in."

I had made my point. Surely there wouldn't be any problem going forward.

Des came in and I got up and helped her to her seat. She held tightly onto my hand.

"Good to meet you, Dr. Ladrin. You come highly recommended."

Des smiled sweetly at her, but her usual magic didn't work. There was no smile in return. This doctor was humorless.

"Thank you," Dr. Ladrin said dryly.

There was an extended pause, then Des spoke again.

"I'm sure that you're surprised that I want all of the medical details given to my husband, but that's my decision." She paused, then shifted gears. "Did my husband tell you that I am trying to choose between a stem cell transplant and your protocol?"

Des may not have known the number of lymph nodes involved or the size of her tumor or the staged number that had been assigned to it, but she did know that her cancer was serious and had gone forward to learn about options for aggressive breast cancer.

"Dr. Pardi," Dr. Ladrin said sternly, "with the size of your tumor and the number of lymph nodes involved, I would not recommend a stem cell transplant. It would be a foolish idea." Then, as if to punctuate her warning, she took off her glasses and looked Des in the eye. "You are at very high risk for it to return."

I had been holding Des's hand the whole time. At that point, I felt her stiffen. Then she pulled her hand away, looked at me, her eyes filled with tears.

Oh, no. This is exactly what I didn't want to happen.

She got up and walked quietly out of the room.

Dr. Ladrin watched as Des left the room, then she turned to me and said curtly, "Your wife is very emotional, Mr. Pardi."

Very emotional! I wanted to wring her neck, but as calmly as I could, I got up, closed the door and walked over to her desk. "Who are you to do that?" I asked. "What right do you have to go against my wife's wishes?"

"Mr. Pardi..."

"How could you say that to her when we specifically requested that no such information be given? Do you realize that you are taking away all of her hope? Do you realize she is entitled to her own coping mechanisms and no one, not even God, has the right to take that away from her? This is how she chooses to cope. She's a person, before she is a patient! It's her right. Who the hell are you to take this away from her?"

"I'm a physician and..."

"Physician? You are a heartless drone and I pity the people who come to see you," I found coming out of my mouth. "You need to learn that it's *people* you're dealing with, and not just cases in a goddamned textbook. I know that your oath is to do no harm, that is what it means to be a physician. You just caused a patient harm. Consider yourself a complete failure as a physician."

I knew I needed to get out of there because I felt intense rage bubbling up, but there was one more thing this doctor had to hear from me. "One day you will be sick - it's inevitable - and I hope you don't experience the pain that you just caused my wife." I looked at her one last time and then walked out. And yes, I slammed the door as I left.

Des was very upset, and I blamed myself. I would have done anything to have spared her that. Maybe I hadn't made it clear enough. Maybe this doctor didn't understand that it was really what Des wanted. I knew one thing, however: it was never going to happen again.

After interviewing five oncologists, we did find the right one - Dr. Steven Samuels, an important doctor at another major hospital - and he got it - all of it. He was extremely knowledgeable and equally as understanding, which we both felt our doctors needed to be. Moreover, he was already doing studies on stem cell transplants, an aggressive treatment Des has spent hours learning about and though considered highly unorthodox at the time, she had nonetheless decided that it was the course she was going to pursue.

"I want to beat this thing," she said to me. "I'm young, I'm strong. My body can handle something really tough."

From what I had been reading, this would be a really rough procedure, but she was looking at it from an educated point of view and I was certainly going to support her decision. We made arrangements to start the necessary pre-procedure chemo right after Christmas.

I'd always loved Christmas, especially Christmas Eve when my family did the traditional Italian thing. My mother and grandmother had always spent hours preparing The Feast of the Seven Fishes: Shrimp, scallops, smelts, calamari, baccala, spaghetti *alle vongole*, and another which I always forget. This year we were missing my Grandmother Fella, who had died the year before, but she was certainly with us in spirit. My brother and his then girlfriend

Maddy were there and despite the issues I had with my father, it was a festive time.

Everyone was so glad to see Des, and even though, to my mother's and father's disappointment, she wasn't "a nice Italian girl," Des had captured their hearts early on in our relationship, and her illness had affected them deeply.

"We're so glad that we can all be together, my mom said, hugging Des. Then my father hugged her too, his eyes a bit misty. Des and I later learned that he had recently been diagnosed with cancer himself - lung cancer that would claim him a year later.

On Christmas Day we went to my in-laws. Without question, their hearts were in the right place, but as much as they tried, the atmosphere seemed gloomy. And how could it not be? Their daughter had just been diagnosed with cancer. She had been diagnosed and operated on in a foreign country. What it must have been like for them to not even kiss their daughter before going into surgery.

Des's mother had prepared a baked ham and, of course, the beer was plentiful. The food was passed, but anxiety blanketed the table.

Then her sister spoke up. "We all feel just horrible that you're so sick."

"We're all just too upset," Des's mother said sadly.

"Well, I'm not upset," Des said, "so why should you be?"

"Breast cancer is dangerous!" her mother blurted out. As a nurse, she was well aware of how devastating cancer could be.

I knew that would rankle Des. She was so intent in putting cancer in a box, compartmentalizing it in her own unique way as being the only way she could cope and move forward with the positivity she was so sure she would need. They needed to engage in what was happening. Des had already made peace with it, but here in front of them, for the first time was their daughter and sister, dealing with cancer.

She snapped at her mother, and later was so sorry that she had. But at the moment, her fear propelled her.

"Well, I've got my PhD in physiology and biophysics, and I'm halfway through medical school, Mom, so I know about that. And you know what?" she continued, looking straight at her mother, "it's OK. "And I'm OK, as long as you don't make a big thing about it. I intend to get rid of this cancer, but what I don't intend to do is to make it the center of my existence. Now let's change the subject."

I could see her mother's eyes well up and so could Des. "Oh, Mom, I'm sorry. Sometimes I forget how this all is affecting you and Dad. It's just that I have to do it my way. Won't you help me and please understand that?"

And of course it was affecting them, but Des desperately needed to do it her way. She had to be in control, had to follow her own path. She felt that is was the only way she could get through it all. She had forewarned me that her family probably would not understand her wanting to "live around the disease" and not focus on it, knowing, of course, they wanted to help – especially since her mother was a nurse. She knew they wanted to talk about it, needed to talk about it, but she couldn't. It was her journey to navigate her way. She simply did not want to talk about her cancer – particularly on a holiday and with me there to protect her. Shielding Des from any kind of negativity, even from loving and well-meaning people, would become an ongoing mission for me.

In the beginning, her mom came to treatments and there was some light and genuine laughter, but then Des started to feel that she was being thrown off her course. And as much as she said she didn't want to read them, her mother, needing to help, continued to send her books and articles about breast cancer. There were even books about positivity. She was doing what she felt was in her daughter's best interests, to be sure, but the way she looked at things was totally different from the way Des did. The same can be said of her father, her sisters and the many other people in her life at that time who cared about her, whether family or friends. Des felt strongly that it was her right to cope with her illness in the way she chose to, and those who didn't, from her point of view, had to be distanced. She didn't realize how much her illness affected those around her, and how much they were hurting, and how much her "cocooning" impacted others. But she firmly believed that the more she focused on it, the less successful she would be in keeping a positive attitude, and keeping a positive attitude was paramount to her. She started relying on me to be her buffer not only between her and her doctors, but also between her and those who loved her. The pressure on me was great and growing every day, and even though I knew it would take its toll in the long run, I was going to stand by her 100 per cent and do what she needed, regardless of the fallout.

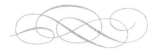

Chapter 15

After spending Christmas Eve and Christmas Day with our respective families, we made our annual December 26 pilgrimage to mid-town Manhattan. We always loved New York during the holiday season, especially between Christmas and New Year's when some of the frenzy, but none of the joy, had diminished. It was wonderful to walk down Fifth Avenue, look in the store windows, experience the rush of tourists and shoppers and stop for a hot chocolate with lots of whipped cream. We especially loved the glittering ball that looked down over 57th Street and Fifth Avenue, and the amazing windows at Bergdorf Goodman, more works of art than commercial displays.

The weather on this day after Christmas was cold but clear and sunny and we enjoyed every minute. Des was as excited as a child, taking in all the holiday sights. One never would have known that on the following day she was going to start chemotherapy in advance of a stem cell procedure. She was so positive about the whole thing, and I knew that, not only did I have to match her mood I also had to feel as positive as well.

"This is a good day," she said with a genuine smile on her face as we went to the hospital. "Today will enable me to get better, to achieve my goal of becoming the best doctor I can be, and to spend a really, really long life with you Mr. Robert Pardi, Jr."

I squeezed her hand. "Yes," I said. "Yes, it is a good day!"

We reported to the chemotherapy section of a major New York hospital's oncology division on that day, and then every three weeks after that for six months, where Des cheerfully submitted to having a line inserted into a vein and having powerful chemicals flushed into her bloodstream and dealing with it as though it were nothing more than a minor inconvenience.

Like most New York hospitals, this one was a huge, imposing place, with a labyrinth of wings and long, seemingly endless corridors. After a couple of wrong turns, we found the oncology department and when we walked into the chemo room, three of the four chairs were already occupied. One woman, middle-aged and somewhat frail, was dozing, her turbaned head lilting to the side. A second woman, 40ish, pleasant-looking and a bit more robust, was sitting upright, staring off into space, an unopened book in her lap. Her full head of reddish-brown hair just grazed her shoulders. A third woman, also 40ish, but thin and gaunt, was working a crossword puzzle. She had very short, salt and pepper hair - almost a buzz cut - and huge hoops, which had a kind of defiance about them, hung from her ears.

Des and I both smiled and said "hello" and I stood guard as the nurse settled Des in.

"I'll be right back with your meds," she said cheerfully as she walked toward the door.

I quickly caught up with her.

"Excuse me, Ms... Ms..."

"Saatvika. Just call me Vee," she said, with the sweetest, most caring tone in her voice.

"Vee, thank you. I'm Robert Pardi, Desiree Pardi's husband."

"I assumed as much," she said, with a big, friendly smile. "Now what can I do for you?"

"Did Dr. Samuels's office tell you about my wife's protocol?" I was already talking the word-specific language of cancer.

"Of course they did," she laughed and patted me on the arm. "She'll be getting Adriamycin, Cytoxan and Taxol. I think she chose the order herself, if I understood correctly, right?"

"Yes. Yes, she did. She wanted the acronym to be A.C.T." I answered. "But she doesn't want to hear about any of the side effects."

Vee looked puzzled. "Well, now," she said, looking at me over the top of tortoise-shell half glasses, "did she already read about them as well?"

"Actually, Vee, she didn't. She does not want to anticipate any side effects. It makes it easier for her to cope that way."

Vee thought for a moment. "You know, she may have a point there. Never thought of it that way." And then she smiled. "Not to worry, Mr. Pardi. I'll take good care of her."

Vee's big, open smile reassured me, and I impulsively kissed her on the cheek. "You're a sweetheart," I said. She patted me on the back and went on down the hall. I hoped that all the medical personnel we would be encountering would be as understanding.

When I returned to the chemo room, Des, in typical fashion, was laughing and bringing the others along on the ride.

"Didn't you just love that Will Smith movie?" Ever the optimist, Smith's "Pursuit of Happiness" was a favorite of hers. The older, frail woman, who I later learned was named Dora, preferred "Life is Beautiful," the touching WWII drama that won Italian actor Roberto Benigni an Oscar and made him an international star.

Rona, the woman with the thick hair - which, I later learned, was a sign that she was just beginning her treatments and not yet in the hair loss phase - liked "Shakespeare in Love."

"Wasn't Gwyneth Paltrow just wonderful?" she asked, wistfully. The group was pretty much in agreement with that.

They each had their favorites and thanks to Des, who was always the ringleader, they were able to take their minds off their very real medical problems and find some joy in laughter and companionship.

The hospital had done their best to make the atmosphere as pleasant as possible. The chairs were large and comfortable, the room was painted a pale peach and there were soft, pleasing pictures on the walls. And that awful medicinal smell that usually permeates hospital air, seemed to have been conquered.

Over the many weeks Des had chemo, the group was basically the same. The women were all on strict schedules. Sometimes she was successful in engaging them in conversation, but there were other times when she wasn't. We quickly learned that dealing with cancer and all that it entails was different for just about everyone.

Two of the other women were breast-cancer patients - each a number in the one-in-eight tally of US women who would suffer with the disease at some point during their lifetime. Each had eventually lost her hair, and each dealt with it in a different way. The newest woman in the group, Robin, a forty-five-year-old, had chosen to face the world with a bald head. I had never seen a woman with a bald head before, and I thought she was very brave. On some levels, the sight of her was shocking but, on another level, it was a revelation. It made me look past the obvious and I saw a beauty in her that didn't depend on a head full of hair. I hoped her husband told her that she looked beautiful. I don't know, because he never came to the hospital.

Two of the other women were married, but their husbands never showed up to lend support either. I never understood that. Maybe they didn't have any flexibility at work. Or maybe they just couldn't handle it. Or maybe the women didn't want them there. This was not the case with Des and it certainly never occurred to me not to be there with her. Her fellow patients called us "The Twins" because if they saw the one, they would surely see the other.

Robin's grown daughter came with her each time, and Dora had a friend who I saw from time to time. The women usually did their best to be cheerful, but I could see the fear in their eyes. I was frightened for them - and I certainly was frightened for Des.

As up and positive as she was, the prospect of losing her hair terrified her. At the time, pretty much all the drugs used for breast cancer caused the patient to lose her hair. Des's hair was beautiful, long and thick, and although born blonde, as she grew into puberty, it had turned brown. By the time she was a teenager, she chose to become blonde again, and although I had never seen her with brown hair, I thought that nature must somehow have made a mistake to let her hair darken because blonde hair looked so perfect on her.

"I'm going to look so horrible when I lose my hair," she said, snuggled up next to me that night. "What if I have a funny shaped head? You won't love me anymore."

"That's ridiculous! Of course, I will."

She laughed nervously and I laughed with her, but I knew it would be difficult for her. And when she decided to get her hair cut in stages so that the final loss of it wouldn't be quite so traumatic, I fully supported her decision. We didn't discuss it, but I was really concerned that once all of her hair would be gone, the old insecurities that she had fought so hard to conquer would return.

At the time, I was struggling more and more with the idea of quitting my job in The Emirates and coming home for good. As I pretty much suspected, Des, however, wouldn't hear of it.

"No!" she had said firmly that night before the first round of chemo, while we were at a neighborhood diner having some hot chocolate. "You're so good at what you do – and you like it. Why should you have to give it up? Plus Snoopy, I love Abu Dhabi."

"I am going to do what I need to do and finish med school" she said, resolve burning in her eyes. "And you need to do what is right for you. We can't let it change our lives any more than it has to. The only impact cancer is going to have on me is that it will help me be a better doctor. I am going to learn from this experience and learn from it big time."

She put her arm through mine and pulled me close. "And you, Mr. World-Class Investment Guru, are going to stay put in Abu Dhabi. You are *not* going to change anything - except, of course, when you're here with me for chemo, and when you're looking after me when I'm back in Abu Dhabi with you!"

As impossible as it may sound, after each round of chemo, Des made the trip to Abu Dhabi with me and stayed until it was time for us to go back to New York for the following round. Dr. Samuels, her oncologist, knew how important it was for her to be with me and he sanctioned it, just as long as she wore a protective mask on the flights. Being able to join me in Abu Dhabi was key to Des's recuperation. And he understood that. The label "Palliative Care" may not have been stamped on that decision, but looking back, it's clear that not only was he embracing the philosophy in how he was practicing medicine, certainly insofar as Des was concerned, but by making these choices, she was clearly paving the way to making the career choice that she ultimately did.

"Patients should be able to have more say about how their illnesses are treated and what's important to them," Des said. "Patients should have their dignity. They should have a say in how they want to live their lives while they are sick. It should be people before patients, Robert. Why haven't we been able to make that happen? We are so fortunate to have Dr. Samuels. He understands this. Anybody else would probably have given me an absolute 'no' to traveling to Abu Dhabi. More doctors need to wake up. There has to be change - real change. Patients have to be viewed as human beings...real people and not just patients."

Neither of us realized it at that moment, but Desiree Pardi, the palliative care crusader, was being born. And what I probably didn't realize, at that moment, was how very difficult it must have been for Des to stay that strong and not show me the fear she must have had. She did that for me, not only then, but all throughout her illness. My love for her was matched only by her love for me.

My supervisors at the Investment Authority were extremely understanding of my need to fly back to the States every three weeks and, with the generous vacation time my contract afforded, I was able to work it out - even though any savings we thought we could accumulate were eaten up by the flights. Knowing that none of what was happening was dragging down my career made Des happy. She was so proud of my success and was my biggest cheerleader, buoying me up and discounting any doubts I may have had. At that point however, my career was the last thing I cared about. Des's cure was the only thing that really mattered to me. The only thing.

We toasted Des's resolve, then went home and made love. That part of our life together had been so important to both of us before Des got sick and we wanted so much for it to stay the same. But after the mastectomy it had changed and, in all likelihood, would continue on that downward slope until Des was free and clear and able to feel whole again.

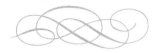

Chapter 16

S tandard rounds of chemo were a necessary prelude to the autologous stem cell transplant which is when a patient's stem cells are harvested from their bone marrow - treated to free them of cancer and then reintroduced to the body. It is designed to kill off all the cancer cells and create an environment in which the stem cells would re-populate with only healthy cells, beef up the immune system and in doing so, help the body ward off a recurrence.

During the process, the patient's body is practically brought as close to death as possible through high-dose chemotherapy. For me, it was an absolutely terrifying prospect. It was rough - really rough - with all the attendant weakness, nausea and vomiting, but Des was consistently cheerful and never once complained. On the contrary, she said more than once, that her goal was to be healthy and that this treatment was matching her goal. Never once was her resolve to go forward with the transplant lessened.

I, on the other hand, walked around with a perpetual knot in my stomach, reciting a silent mantra of "it's got to work, it's got to work" that fell somewhere between a wish and a prayer. How could this have happened to such a healthy, vital girl who had so much to look forward to and so much to contribute? I just couldn't understand it or accept it.

When I was first told about the severity of Des's cancer, I was informed that the odds were 80 per cent that it would come back and that she would most likely be dead in three years, so when the post-chemo tests showed that Des was completely free of malignancy, I was not totally relieved. How could I be? And how could Des? Although she did not know all the specifics of her situation, she'd still had several years of scientific education under her belt, and as much as I had tried to protect her from the information, the leap to conclusion had to have been there. Deep down, she had to have known and was doing her best to be strong for me. What a burden that must have been.

But Des, always so thorough in everything she did, wanted to max out on whatever was available in the known cancer arsenal - no matter how difficult the procedure. And the stem cell transplant certainly fell into that category. This was in 1999 and the prevailing medical wisdom at the time was that these procedures might be effective in preventing recurrence in high-risk breast cancer patients, with the operative word being "might." As had quickly become my habit, I read everything I was able to find about the procedure and it seemed beyond difficult to me. Even more important, its efficacy was in no way proven. Des, however, was determined. Years later, the results of these studies showed that it did not at all prolong life or reduce the risk of cancer returning.

"I'm going to nuke this thing!" she said emphatically, shaking her head. I could only smile and shake my head 'yes' with her, because Des was resolute and that was good enough for me.

After she finished the four months of chemotherapy, we went back to Abu Dhabi where Des got a welcome respite from hospitals and chemo. She quickly got into a rhythm of relaxation, enjoying the Gulf and the beach resorts and having dinners with friends. She was so happy and upbeat, no one would have guessed what she had just endured - and what she had ahead of her.

But after three months, it was time to go back to the States, check into the hospital and get ready for the transplant. At first, Des was put into a room with another patient. I didn't quite understand that, since what I had read indicated that the less contact patients had with others, the better. Des was OK with it, but when I saw some dirt on the floor in the shared bathroom that was it for me. I didn't care if they had to build an extension to the hospital, Des was going to get a private room.

There were none available, I was emphatically told - first by the on-duty nurse, then by the head nurse. The resident, too, was negative. Yet somehow I was going to get her a private room or die trying. After much insistence Dr. Samuels was finally able to make it happen.

The bureaucracy was maddening. During the several months that Des had been undergoing procedures I had been thrust into a whole new world and, for someone who had never spent much time in hospitals, I was quickly getting the hang of how things worked - who to talk to, how to handle them, when to push and when not to. These institutions, I learned, are fiefdoms of power and a miss-step can cost you dearly. I had gone from negotiating with stock and bond traders and corporate executives to steely and sometimes ego-driven medical personnel. I couldn't afford to screw up, or to lose my temper - the latter of which I felt was highly likely. There were times when my self-control was pushed to the limits but I had to keep a lid on it. What was happening was too crucial. I wished I had been more of an insider in the system, and once again I really regretted my decision of many years before not to go to medical school.

There was yet another course of punishing chemotherapy - 24 hours a day for five days. Des's hair came out, once again, and she had just started growing it back, but she didn't let that dampen her positive attitude.

Early on in the treatment, she was seized with an uncontrollable fit of vomiting. Nothing that we had not experienced before but, this time, her body reacted while she was talking to me, and instead of words, I got a huge dose - all over me.

Tears welled up in Des's eyes.

"Robert, oh my God. I am so, so sorry."

"Baby, sorry? You know this is nothing new for me," I said with a big smile, trying to make light of it. "Remember that time in school when we had too many chocolate martinis, not to mention those lethal blue whales, and you unloaded on me?"

But that didn't make her laugh. She looked so forlorn and I wanted so much just to take her in my arms and assure her that it was nothing, but I was a mess and it just would have made matters worse.

So I just kissed her on the forehead - something of which the doctors certainly would have disapproved - and said what was in my heart.

"We are in this together, Baby. You know I would take the chemo for you if I could."

Tears rolled down her face. "I believe you would," she said. "I really do." She smiled and then kind of drifted off, thanks to the sedation that is given along with the chemo in an attempt to make it more tolerable.

I sat by her bed and read to her, and as silly as it may sound, books she had enjoyed from her childhood, such as *Dr. Seuss* and the *Nancy Drew* mysteries and then more serious and interesting works, like the play, *The Glass Menagerie.*

When it came time for them to re-introduce Des's stem cells, the numbers on her charts did not add up, and indications were that the cells might not be hers. If they gave Des the wrong ones, she would die. I couldn't believe it! How could they even think of going forward when everything wasn't 100 per cent? As far as I was concerned, there was no way. I made them pull every last piece of documentation and show me where the mistake had been made. Much of the posting had been done by hand, and, as it turned out, someone had just transposed some numbers.

With stem cells transplants, the patient must be kept totally germ-free. This means the room has to be spotless, visitors sparse and anyone entering the room must be dressed in a virtual Hazmat suit. I was not about to trust that the staff had done a proper job of disinfecting. I know they thought I was nuts but I scrubbed down every part of that room...cleaned the floor on my hands and knees, disinfected everything that could be touched, from the bed rails to the light switches.

And to say that I did not encourage visitors would be putting it mildly. My tense relationship with my in-laws became even more so when I made them stay several feet away from the bed when visiting Des. I know they appreciated that the care I was taking had turned me into a virtual warden, but this was also their daughter whom they loved and were worried sick about. The line was so hard to walk at times, and became even harder as time went on, but I had to my watch. It was the job Des entrusted me to carry out. I knew they were hurting, which was one of the many reasons I was wide-eyed late into the night, but I was just not going to chance anything happening to Des.

Proximity to Des did not extend to me. Even if I had put myself off limits, Des wanted me nearby. I had graduated from husband and lover to patient advocate, medical negotiator and all-around buffer, and as the days went by, those roles took over more and more of my consciousness. Abu Dhabi and the worlds of money and finance could have been on another planet, not just a couple of oceans away. I maintained telephone contact with my office, but I can't imagine I was in any way effective. My focus on business was totally gone, and I doubted even if and when Des were totally recovered, I would ever be able to get it back.

I stayed by Des's bedside for the 21 days she was hospitalized, hardly ever leaving. I was scared and, even though she didn't say so, I knew Des was too. How could she not be? It was my job to allay those fears, and the best way I could do it was just to be there and repeat a mantra with her: "Every day I am getting more and more healthy."

It seemed as though everything went according to the book and Des was just about to be released from the hospital when she developed a fever and realized she had an infection in the insertion site of her port - a small, semi-permanent device that makes receiving infusions easier. On her upper chest, near her clavicle, the port site was red and angry looking. The nurse who had installed the port had apparently not disinfected the site well enough when drawing blood. With Purell dispensers now installed every few feet in hospitals, it's hard to believe that at the end of the 20th century, that kind of thing could have happened. I was beside myself, angry at the staff, and angry at myself. It would never happen again. Not on my watch.

The infection subsided in a couple of days and we went home, but about a week later, Des developed what is called a "neutropenic fever," a temperature spike that sometimes accompanies strong chemo or the procedure that Des had just had. In my extensive reading I had learned that this was a possibly lethal side effect of the transplant. I knew that Des also knew that, and I tried not to panic.

She developed chills and started shaking. I wrapped her in blankets and held her close, but nothing I could do could get her warm.

"You'd better get me to the emergency room, Robert," she said with steely calm. "This is a pretty serious complication."

Serious? From what I had read, it was way beyond serious. It was life threatening. I don't know how she kept so calm, but I knew she was doing it for my benefit, not wanting to upset me.

I thought I would crawl out of my skin by the time the ambulance arrived. In the ER Des was infused with mega-doses of antibiotics and then sent right back to the stem cell transplant unit for several days until she had totally recovered. It seemed surreal to be back there again.

Yet with all she had just been through, Des's spirits were still good. She never veered into "Why me?" territory. Not once. Had it been me, I think I would have been screaming at the top of my lungs. Sometimes when she was dozing, I would just look at her and marvel. My God. This woman I married...her resilience was extraordinary.

I was in a constant battle with myself to stay strong. Sometimes the fear would be paralyzing, but I couldn't allow it to immobilize me. I had to focus and keep going forward.

Des loved board games and I managed to get my hands on some. We played "Life," where reaching old age took on a whole new meaning, and "Candy Land," which even little kids can navigate. But it helped to pass the time and we laughed a lot. And we watched movies. There was a DVD player in the room and I happily endured Des's devotion to "Pretty Woman" and "Auntie Mame." Whatever she wanted to watch was fine with me.

"Don't think too many of my med school classmates have had this kind of hands-on experience!" she said impishly. "I'll do anything to get a jump on them!" Then she laughed again, with her wonderful, girlish laugh and that big, dazzling smile. "I'm going to beat this thing," she said, then corrected herself. "No. I am beating it!"

"Yes you are!" Then I corrected myself: "Yes you *have*!"

She had not one hair on her head but to me she had never looked so beautiful. Yes, my Des was certainly beating it.

Correction: she certainly had beaten it.

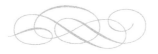

Chapter 17

Des came home and started to regain her strength. I felt like I could breathe again, but the fact that I had totally neglected my job began to gnaw at me. The Investment Authority had been extremely understanding and generous about the time I had taken off but I had been pushing it. My head knew what I had to do. My heart, however, had a different agenda.

"You know, Baby, I can just ditch this job," I said, yet again. "I'll find something here in New York."

That still was not what Des wanted to hear.

"No, Robert," she said, shaking her head. "I am determined that this diagnosis is not going to change our lives. It's just something I have to deal with."

"We," I interjected.

"Yes," she said, "something that *we* have to deal with. Besides, I like the life your job in Abu Dhabi is allowing us to experience a great life." She kissed me on the cheek. "We've gotten me through this procedure, Robert. Our life is good, and now I'm cancer free!"

"Thank God!" I said, squeezing her hand. I couldn't believe the miracle had happened.

To ensure her remission, the doctors had also prescribed six weeks of radiation. I stayed for the first week but then, no matter how much I objected, Des insisted that I return to my job.

"You've really got to go back, Robert," she said. Then a cute, devilish smile crossed her face. "But..." she said, pausing mid-sentence.

I hadn't a clue.

"After I'm finished with the radiation, I'm going to join you in Abu Dhabi!"

I hadn't thought about that possibility at all, but because of all that had happened, Des had missed the deadline for returning to medical school that semester, so why not? Instead of being alone in New York, she could come back with me, relax, spend more time on the beach, which she loved, regain her strength and just, as she put it, "live." What a wonderful idea!

So Des and I cleared it with her doctors, and made plans for her to join me in at the end of the treatment. I returned to Abu Dhabi after that first week of radiation. I had to make sure it all went according to plan and everyone knew that they were never to talk to Des about the specifics of her illness. It was hard to let go of that control. Her mom had told me she was going to watch over Des and honestly, I think that was the best thing for both Des and her mom.

"I'll be fine, just fine and before you know it, I will be back in Abu Dhabi with you going to the Hiltona Beach Club" she said happily. "But you need to get back to work and I need to know life is moving forward for you as well as for us."

On one level, it was good to get back to work and not be so totally immersed in the cancer world. Secure in the knowledge that Des was well and just a few weeks from liberation, I plunged back into research, meetings, and deals - light years from lymph nodes and CT scans and the daily fear that the worst was happening. At last things were good. The worst no longer was happening. Finally.

When Des finished the radiation, it coincided with our wedding anniversary, so of course I flew home. This was a special anniversary - our 10th - and we had so much to be thankful for. We decided to celebrate by renewing our vows and planned a special, intimate dinner with just a few friends. We invited my best friend Dave and his partner Daryl and Des's friend Adira and her husband Alex to be with us and, with the same priest who had originally married us, and in the very same church, we re-dedicated ourselves to one another.

Des, with her nearly bald head and simple dress, was as beautiful that day as she had been the first time around with flowing, blond hair and fairy-tale princess gown. We had been through some really rough patches, but we were so grateful and positive and so much looking forward to the years ahead. The doctors had assured me that Des had done remarkably well and, while there were no guarantees, she was presently free of cancer. My wife was well, we were together and we had our whole future ahead of us.

A few days after our wonderful celebration, Des flew back to Abu Dhabi with me. She re-took to her life there with relish. She regained her strength and never seemed happier, going after the days with energy and excitement. She started every morning at the gym, spent a few hours keeping up to date on her medical reading - joined by the parakeets who nested right outside our window - took Spanish and belly dancing lessons, read spy novels and even tried her hand at cooking again.

"I just love being your wife!" she said with boundless enthusiasm as she tried - with no great success, I may add - to turn out some not-too-complicated dinners. Cooking proved yet again to be her nemesis, so we were regulars at the little café around the corner from our apartment.

Des had to have her blood tested regularly, so once a week we went to a clinic on the outskirts of Abu Dhabi where they took specimens and faxed the results to Dr. Samuels back in the States. Des never seemed anxious while we waited the several days for the results to come back. A simmering level of fear never left me, however, and I did everything I could to mask it. We had beaten the cancer, and that's the way we treated it. Des was just on a well-earned hiatus from years of school, and things would return to normal in just a few months.

Des had always loved the sun and the beach, so I surprised her with a membership to the best beach club in Abu Dhabi. While excited about it, she was concerned about how she looked.

"How can I go in the water with the prosthesis?" she asked, referring to the fake breast she generally wore to balance out her chest. "What if the damn thing pops out in the water? I can see it now," she laughed, "like some jellyfish floating in the surf. Some kid will probably try to spear it!"

She was laughing, but I knew how difficult this was for her. She had always looked so drop-dead gorgeous in a bathing suit - especially a bikini. I did some investigating and found there were bathing suits designed for women with mastectomies and I ordered a few for her.

She was thrilled. "Snoopy, you think of everything!"

I wasn't sure I succeeded in thinking of everything, but I sure as hell tried.

The suits looked great on her and she went swimming nearly every day. Short, light brown curls were growing on her head and she got some color in her face. She glowed, and the world seemed like a good place once again.

We met for lunch every day at the nearby café. Sometimes we lingered there and other times we went home for a siesta. As in most middle eastern countries, the mid-day heat in Abu Dhabi encourages siestas and business hours are structured to accommodate them.

Des's Spanish class was in the early evening at a center not far from the apartment. That worked out well because office hours started up again at 5 and continued until 8. She'd go to her class and then I would pick her up afterward and we would take a walk along the water and then have dinner. It was an easy lifestyle, and Des flourished.

One afternoon she called and said she wasn't going to class, that evening. Could I pick her up at home, instead, to go to dinner?

"Are you feeling OK?" I asked, as a rush of worry coursed through my body.

"Oh, I'm fine," she said cheerfully. "Nothing like that. I just don't feel like going to class. No bigee."

I didn't think she would keep anything from me, at this point, but I was hard pressed to stay in the office until closing time. At eight I rushed home and as I was walking down the hall towards the apartment, I heard middle eastern music - not all that unusual in greater Abu Dhabi, of course, but definitely so on our floor which was rented primarily to westerners like us. One was more likely to hear U2 or Coldplay, but this was the sound of ouds and riqs and when I opened the door to the apartment, the strong aroma of nutmeg, ginger and clove wafted over me. The lights were low and there were candles all around and there was Des, eyes rimmed in Cleopatra black coal, gold coins dangling from the scarf wrapped around her head, dressed in flame red harem pants and a halter top. She was gyrating, slowly, rhythmically, sensuously - my little Irish girl from Long Island - doing as good a job as the world-class belly dancers we had seen in clubs in Morocco.

"Come on in," Robert, she cooed.

I didn't need much coaxing. She had ordered a middle eastern feast and we sat on the floor, as is the custom, and enjoyed mou-jadara - lentil puree with onion - fresh thyme salad with arugula, rice and tomato-stuffed grape leaves, grilled sardines with dandeli-on greens, and chicken livers with pomegranate. It was a feast, and when it was finished, we made love and neither one of us allowed the altered state of her body to interfere.

"Come on Robert. Boobette wants some attention!"

Shortly after the mastectomy, we had taken to calling Des's remaining breast her "boobette." She was so cute and remarkably light-hearted about it. When you hear some medical people say that attitude is so important, they couldn't be more on the mark. Des's spirit was indomitable - and I know that helped add years to her life.

During my time in Abu Dhabi, I had become friendly with a couple of other Americans who worked at the Investment Authority and it was fun to hang out with them. It was good to be with fellow travelers in a sea of middle-easterners. Jack and his Swiss wife Angelica, who adored cats and had a house filled with them, Chuck and his wife Alice, who were from the east coast and had had a hard time adjusting to the Middle East, and Mannie, a New Yorker with no wife and no likely prospects.

In the Emirates, liquor can only be served in restaurants that are attached to hotels, and we had long since found all the good ones. When Des arrived, it was great. The guys and their wives were totally captivated by her and her seemingly boundless zest for life. Cancer was never a topic of discussion.

But at the end of the day, it was Des and me, which is not to say that I hadn't made any really close friends. One of the closest relationships I had back then - and still do today - is with my friend Laith Hameed, the son of a British mother and an Iraqi father. We became fast friends and I grew close to his parents, as well. Of course, they fell in love with Des and the five of us spent a great deal of time together. Laith was as free as a bird, back then, but today he is a proud husband and father. I know Des would have loved seeing him married, holding his baby boy in his arms.

Des also got along very well with my Emirati friends Raashid, Najib and Mustapha, all of whom worked at the Abu Dhabi Investment Authority with me. But it was my colleague Khaled, who had treated us to first-class airfare some months back when we needed to get back to the States after the mastectomy, who really fell for her - as Des did for him - and, as the years went by, would prove to be an amazingly loyal and generous friend as well as close business associate.

But most of all, Des and I had each other. We were a corporation of two and our mission was believing in the future. If Des didn't think her future would be cancer-free, she never let on. As for me, I couldn't allow negative thoughts. When they crept in, as they often did, I expedited them as best I could. Des's plans were in place. She would return to med school the following year, finish her last two years, do her internship and then a residency, most likely in oncology. She had planned to have a career in internal medicine, but her experience as a cancer patient challenged her decision.

"I'm thinking about changing direction and specializing in oncology. What use is all of this personal experience if I don't share it?", she said one afternoon. What neither of us knew then was that it would be the fledgling field of Palliative Care, the precepts of which had been burrowing themselves deeply into her consciousness, that would later capture her heart and inspire her to put her considerable medical knowledge and talent in dealing so effectively with patients to such good use in the future.

I, too, needed a change in direction, but my own path was not clear. The Abu Dhabi position was supposed to be a stop-over. It was never intended to be the route to the rest of my life. The original plan, before Des got sick, was for me to go back to school and get the credits necessary for me to teach. I already had earned my master's in finance, so it wouldn't have involved that much time, but things had taken such a huge shift in focus and direction, and our financial needs had grown in ways that we had never anticipated, that I had to put those plans on hold. I really needed to earn money, so I had a lot of thinking to do.

We returned to Abu Dhabi and picked up where we had left off. Work was good, and we had just about settled back into our routine when we learned that my father had died from the lung cancer that had been diagnosed the year before. Our differences aside, the reason I was not present during his illness was Des's situation. Ironically, it was Des who had been more sympathetic to him - not so much because she, too, was a cancer patient, but more because that's who she was. She had empathetic qualities way beyond the norm - a quality so necessary to the palliative care specialty she would go on to embrace.

To be honest, I don't know how I felt when my father passed. There had always been something so negative between us and I grew to dislike him as a person. The truth is we had never gotten along. For as long as I could remember, it was as though my very being was an assault to his sense of himself...kind of like "how could I have a son like this?" I wish I could say that it had been different, but it hadn't. But, regardless of my dislike and lack of admiration for the man, he was my father and I did need to be there for my mother and brother. So, we hoped on a plane back to New York for the funeral. It was the right thing to do, but frankly, I had no desire to.

As much as Des enjoyed being in Abu Dhabi and what she referred to and we both laughed at - spending her time being "an ordinary housewife" - she was eager to put her plans into place for her re-entry and return to school. But there was something she wanted to do before that. Because her pre-mastectomy breasts had been so big, she felt enormously lop-sided and decided to have the other breast removed as well. Although she didn't say so, I'm sure that fears of the cancer showing up in the second breast played a big part in her decision, but what she talked about was her comfort level...her body image. It would help her feel normal, and that would help her cope. The better she coped, she explained, the more easily she could pursue her goals. Once again, without putting a name to it, Des was making decisions that were purely palliative care choices.

So in February 2000, Des had her second breast removed. She was characteristically strong and resolute about the procedure and its aftermath. We were both relieved that the results of the tests that were done on the breast were negative, but Des felt strongly that she had made the right decision.

After the surgery, she had reconstruction on both breasts. The surgeon took tissue from her groin and used it to fashion nipples, and when the bandages were removed, we both cried. The results were everything we could have hoped for. Her new, modestly sized breasts said "beautiful, healthy woman" and a bright new chapter was about to be written.

Chapter 18

E ven though Des insisted that I should stay put, it was becoming clear to me that I had to get back to New York. Not so much *had* to as *wanted* to. Des was doing well, looking forward to returning to med school, and I needed to lock in something for the future. My colleague and now good friend, Khaled, wanted to start his own investment business in Dubai. He was Western educated, had the resources to back him, and we developed an unwavering trust for each other during my years in Abu Dhabi. One day he told me he wanted me to be his partner. It was an intriguing proposition. When he agreed that part of the deal would be my opening a New York branch, it seemed like the perfect solution. Des would be back at med school in New York, and we could be together again all the time, and not just on vacation or on the sick leave we hoped Des would never need again. It was time to move on to the next phase of our lives.

When Des had come to live in Abu Dhabi the first time, in 1998, we had let go of our old studio apartment. I really loved that place and really hadn't agreed with that decision, but Des said she didn't want to hold on to the past and would want to start fresh when she returned to New York with a spacious grown-up apartment with real furniture and not just a walk-up with a Murphy bed. When she was diagnosed we scrambled to try and get our old place back, because it had only been a few weeks after we gave it up. No chance, but we had a good relationship with our landlord, who owned a few properties in the area, and he offered us what he described as "a really nice large studio" in a doorman building just down the street. He had always been good to us, so we trusted him and took the apartment sight unseen. It proved to be a great decision. It was bright and sunny and just what we needed going forward.

Des was back in the swing of things at Mount Sinai and I was traveling back and forth from my new job in Dubai. I was doing outreach for Evolvence, the firm Khaled and I started together, making contacts and sourcing out possible investments. It was work I enjoyed, and it was great being back in New York on a regular basis, close to our old haunts and the familiar energy of the city. Before long, we were ordering pizza from Ray's, hanging out at Jimmy's and getting back into the swing of things.

Things were going well, or so I thought, but as the months went by, Des seemed to shrink more and more into herself, and even though repeated scans showed that she was cancer free, she had a nagging, dark feeling that the cancer would return.

"I can't help but feel that the Sword of Damocles is hanging over me," Des said more than once, and her sunny optimism gave way to a deep depression.

She had gone through so much with such strength and courage. I hated seeing her in this state. I did everything I could to help her out of it, but as I was trying to boost her up, I was fighting big battles with my own fear.

I was able to arrange my own work schedule, so we had lots of quality time together, but nothing seemed to help. I asked her oncologist if he could recommend a therapist for Des. When he saw how depressed she was, he agreed.

"I really, really, really don't want to go," she protested, her usual bright smile now long gone from her face. "I just know I am not going to like it."

But Dr. Samuels and I were able to persuade Des that it was the best thing to do, and he arranged for her to see a psychiatrist. She went kicking and screaming, not wanting to rehash the demons she thought she had long since conquered or, of course, discuss the illness she had so adamantly tucked away in a corner. She had had cancer, and the possibility of it returning was very real.

But over several sessions, Des begrudgingly started to see the therapy's value. The psychiatrist prescribed Lexapro and Well-butrin and the drugs, in combination with the therapy, pulled her out. But even though, at one point, much earlier, Des had actually thought about becoming a psychiatrist herself, she some-how thought of it as a negative that she had to see a "god-damned shrink!" When I reminded her that at one time she had thought about being a "god-damned shrink," she didn't even see the humor in it. That's how far she had sunk. But when a year of therapy was over, she laughed heartily at it.

"I'm pretty sure I'd rather specialize in internal medicine and disciplines related to oncology, at this point, rather than be a shrink, but I can sure use this experience to help me help my patients in the future. Imagine if doctors really took the time to know about and understand the anxieties their patients were going through!"

Years later, of course, as a leading practitioner of palliative care, she would go on to use all of her psychological skills to understand and help so many struggling with the pain and despair caused by many illnesses but most especially by cancer, the disease Pulitzer Prize winning author Dr. Siddhartha Mukherjee so aptly titled "The Emperor of All Maladies."

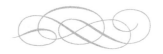

Chapter 19

In August of that year, Des went back to med school and it was as if she were reborn. Her spirits were up, once again, and she threw herself into it with all the resolve she had before breast cancer entered our lives. One of the reasons re-entering was such a positive experience was Dr. Suzi Rose, a gifted gastroenterologist and the Senior Vice Dean for Medical Education at The Perelman School of Medicine at the University of Pennsylvania. At the time, Dr. Rose was the Associate Dean of Student Affairs at Mount Sinai, and she was extraordinarily helpful in arranging Des's schedule so that she could attend classes and take care of her medical needs and do it in a way that made Des comfortable. In order to cope, Des preferred that her situation not be brought to the attention of other students - and it wasn't. Everything was arranged seamlessly, and Des was so grateful to Dr. Rose. She was a blessing.

Other than the scans she had on a regular basis, the only other reminder that Des was a cancer survivor was the new fashion statement she made wearing scrubs, the light blue shirts and pants worn by senior med students and residents. Because the armholes are loose, Des had to wear a t-shirt under her top to camouflage the scars from her surgeries and the special bra she wore due to her breast reconstruction. It was against Mount Sinai's regulations but there was no way they were going to say "no" to someone who had such a great academic track record, had gone through so much and was so well liked and admired by all her classmates and instructors.

By this time, I had totally relocated to New York and would just be making occasional trips back to the Middle East. And aside from Des's long hours of school and studying, our lives were almost normal. We did nights out with friends and paid visits to both of our families, although the visits with Des's parents were still strained and she didn't want to see them all that often, because she was always afraid her mother would want to talk about her health or give her cancer care books, something Des was adamant about not discussing. Although her mother surely had Des's welfare at heart, and needed to feel she was helping as a mother would need to, they were just not on the same page. Des and I, however, were more bonded than ever. We had come through a long, dark tunnel and were still very much in love.

Every New Yorker remembers where they were on that cloudless, warm, sunny morning of September 11, 2001. I was scheduled to go to a breakfast meeting at Windows on the World in the Twin Towers. As it turned out, I never went. I was one of the lucky ones - and I have my mother to thank for that. She had been after me for weeks to paint her dining room. I had put it off several times, but on that morning, almost on a whim, I decided to skip the meeting and go to Long Island and take care of it.

I went down into the subway to go to Penn Station. We had barely left the station when the train stopped dead in the tunnel. It was rush hour and the train was packed and hot. There was no announcement over the loudspeaker and no one knew what was going on. The car was pretty quiet for a while, then people started to talk, some nervously and too loudly. As the time went on, a couple of people got really anxious about being stuck. The anxiety spread till you could feel it all around, like some virus waiting to ravage you. Some people started to panic, and the fear spread. With great difficulty, I was doing all I could to stay calm. Finally, after more than an hour, the train advanced to the next station and we all got out. It wasn't a minute too soon.

When we hit the outside air, we learned the unimaginable from people on the street. We were stunned - and terrified. Many were frantic. It was impossible to check on loved ones because cell phones weren't working. People started screaming. "My brother!" "Oh my God. My husband works there." A woman collapsed sobbing. "My son, my son." I was one of several people who helped her up. One woman, a total stranger, volunteered to stay with her and help to get her home. There were lots of good Samaritans that day.

Aside from my horror at the news, I was anxious to reach Des and let her know I was all right. I hadn't told her about my change in plans, so she must have thought I was caught in Tower One, where the meeting I was scheduled to attend was being held. I started walking up town and tried repeatedly to reach her from pay phones along the way, but the lines were jammed. Finally, after two hours, I was able to get through.

"Robert, you're alive! I just knew it, I knew it. I could feel you were ok. Thank God...thank God!"

I could hear the sobs of joy.

"I knew you would be OK. I just knew. I could feel you."

"I was lucky, Des," I said, my voice cracking. "So lucky that I had decided to change my plans and go to Long Island instead."

"You were lucky Robert," Des said, still sobbing. "*We* were lucky...so lucky. Thank God..."

Neither one of us wanted to hang up, but Des couldn't talk for more than a moment. Duty called.

"I love you...love you so much, Robert. You know that, don't you?"

"Of course..."

"And thank God you are all right, and I can't believe I actually have to hang up but you know I've gotta go, now."

Of course she did. Every possible medical professional - students included - was on ER duty that day, anticipating a huge influx of survivors to treat for burns, inhalation, broken limbs or trauma. Sadly, as we all know, there were few patients to treat in the aftermath of the horror our nation will never forget. The survivors numbered very few.

I told Des I loved her – more than once. Then I hung up and laughed until I practically cried. I had been so lucky...so very, very lucky.

I continued on my way home uptown. The streets were filled and everyone was incredulous at the news. Restaurants and coffee shops were jammed with people not enjoying food and drink, but just needing to be with people...seeking comfort in the company of others.

It was very warm that day, and I was drenched in sweat by the time I got to our apartment. Des wasn't there, of course, and when she finally got home, hours later, she grabbed me and held onto me for what seemed like forever. We couldn't believe our good fortune. I think that was probably the last time that Des didn't know exactly where I was at every moment of the day or night, and I never minded it one bit. I was so grateful I had decided to paint my mom's dining room, that day, and so grateful that Des was alive and well and doing exactly what she had planned to do before our lives were invaded by cancer.

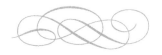

Chapter 20

On May 10, 2002, Des graduated from medical school. "Aside from the day I married the greatest guy in the world," she told everyone who would listen, "this is the happiest day of my life!"

The smile on her face was matched only by the smile on mine. My wife, this amazing woman, not only had gotten a PhD in physiology and biophysics, now she had graduated from medical school as well, and all accomplished with the highest honors - including election to the prestigious Alpha Omega Alpha Honor Society - and all fought for and won against inconceivable odds. Extraordinary!

Her parents and my mom came to the ceremony at Mount Sinai and we went out for lunch afterwards. We were all so proud of Des! The conversation was light and it was pleasant, but Des and I were both anxious to get through it and get home because we were leaving for a trip later that afternoon.

Des loved seeing new places and trying new things, and we had traveled so much during our years together, so it came as no surprise that to celebrate her graduation, she wanted to go on yet another trip.

"Let's go to the beach," she said. "Palm Beach? Delray?"

But I had another idea. I was always trying to come up with fun, new things to do that Des would like. I had read about dolphins and how there was much speculation about their healing powers.

"Swimming with the dolphins!" she said with the wide-eyed enthusiasm of a kid anticipating her first trip to Disney World. "They are soooooo cute - and did you know? They have healing powers."

I smiled, having read that many believed that to be true.

"Snoopy, I love you! This is the best idea!"

Well, I wasn't quite convinced that just being with dolphins in their energy pathways could cure everything from autism to cancer, as some people believed. If that were really true, half the free world would be invading their waters. I did agree, however, that dolphins were kind of cute and I knew their natural habitat was warm water. Des would love that, and the warm water part sounded good to me.

I had done my research and learned that one of the best places for dolphin swimming was near the Club Med in the Bahamas. I anticipated a wild, swinging scene, but this Club Med was family friendly and entirely wholesome. It was terrific, as it turned out, and I ended up really liking it. The beach and water were gorgeous, there was plenty of good food and drink, and we met lots of fun people. But it was Des and the dolphins that made that trip.

The dolphin sanctuary was not far from the resort and we were taken there by a team of dolphin specialists. The huge pool was set in the ocean and several dolphins romped in the water, jumping up and down, twirling about and showing off their best moves. With a tee shirt over her bathing suit - Des had been instructed to shield her chest from the sun since the radiation - Des slid into the water. She walked over to one dolphin that seemed to have his eye on her - perhaps because that day she was the only adult in the small group made of autistic and challenged kids. Des patted him on the nose and he seemed to like that. Then she drew her hand along the length of his body, and he liked that too. A couple of other dolphins vied for her attention. She swam alongside them, dove and cruised with them, and when they made their funny, squeaking sounds, Des squeaked right back. The kids all liked that and there was a lot of squeaking at that point. It was sweet seeing them all having such fun.

Then the first dolphin nestled in. He and Des made noises at each other then, taking a cue from one of the instructors, she took hold of the dolphin's tail and they took off. Let me tell you, Nascar has nothing on these guys! They are fast, but Des stayed on and had the ride of her life.

Along with the kids' parents, I took loads of photos. Des did a great job of playing with the children and didn't seem to mind being the only adult. She liked kids. We both did, but having children just wasn't in the cards.

At one point earlier on, Des did find herself pregnant, even though she had been on the pill. It was during her first year of PhD studies and she didn't say anything to me until just a few weeks into it, when she had a miscarriage.

"I must have forgotten to take a pill," she said to me with the saddest look on her face, "but I guess we don't have to worry about that now." She paused. "Are you upset about this?" she asked me.

I wasn't sure how to respond. I thought about all we had gone through and how much more difficult it would have been had we had a child. "Baby, how could I be upset after all you've been through fighting for your life – our life together?" Frankly, I was happy that there were just the two of us. I was ambivalent about children, at best, because of the way I had grown up, but if that's what Des wanted, I know I would have gone along with it. I know she liked kids. She so enjoyed being an aunt to her sister's little girl, and later on to my brother's daughter, but parenting a child full time was something else, and with all her years of schooling ahead and the way our living style evolved, it just never happened. We were so close and so many times we had talked about how fulfilled we were just being "us" - a corporation of two. Then, when all the chemo put her in pre-mature menopause, having children became a moot point.

But that day we weren't discussing life choices. Des was happy and smiling and enjoying a starring role with a half a dozen laughing kids. I loved seeing her seizing the joy of the moment - something she knew how to do better than just about anyone I have ever known, then or since. She was my teacher and guide about pure, unadulterated joy. She radiated it. Through all her trials, Des managed, every day, to still my heart and take my breath away. Thinking of her today, she still does...

Shortly after that, Des started her internship in the Department of Medicine at New York Presbyterian Hospital/Weill Cornell. "I feel like I'm on top of the world!" she repeated as she left for work every morning. After all the years of studying, hard work and beyond impossible health challenges, she was a working doctor!

At that point, we had moved, yet again - this time to a really nice apartment in a high rise that was owned by the hospital. Des became friends with a number of other interns, at that time, including some young doctors who have gone on to important careers throughout the United States in many areas of medicine, including psychiatry, pulmonary care, and oncology. Among them was Lauren Schwartz, now an award-winning gastroenterologist practicing in Manhattan, with whom she formed an old-fashioned, "best-friend" bond that was a source of exceptional mutual support and comfort as the years went by. We frequently socialized with these medical friends, their spouses and significant others, and the company was good. For the longest time, Des did not share the information with them that she was a recovering cancer patient - and they had no idea: she was so vibrant, healthy looking and full of life! She was doing well, and life was wonderful.

Des spent lots of her spare time - such as it was - on the internet. With her intellectual curiosity, she was always trolling for something about history, or architecture or the latest novels she could devour. She was also a huge Oprah Winfrey fan. She found Oprah very inspirational and appreciated what a great help she was to many people. One day when she was checking Oprah's website, Des saw that the Oprah show was looking for candidates who were graduating from high school "against all odds."

"Look at this, Snoopy," she said, calling me over to the screen. "Too bad they're confining it to high school students. I'd love to be on that show!"

The minute Des was out of the house, I logged back on to the Oprah site, jotted down the information and got to work. I sent a really persuasive email to the producers. As far as I was concerned, no one had beaten more odds than Des. I followed up on the phone and I was able to convince them to include her. I was thrilled and couldn't wait until she got home that evening so I could tell her.

"What?" she asked when she saw me with a huge grin on my face. I was bursting to give her the news.

"Oh, well...just something you'll like." I paused for a little dramatic emphasis. "No. I take that back. Something you'll *really* like!"

"A dog!" she exclaimed wide-eyed. "You got us a dog!"

We couldn't take Dollar$ with us to Abu Dhabi so we "loaned" him to my father when we were both in Abu Dhabi. He was sick with lung cancer, at that point, and Des felt having the dog around would be good for him. When my father succumbed to his cancer, Des's friend Adira took Dollar$.

We were never really sure what had happened, but one day we got a message that Dollar$ had died. Des was very broken up and I promised her that when the time was right, we would get another dog.

"A dog! You got us another dog! Where is he?" She turned and started toward the bedroom. "Bet he's in there!"

"No, sweetie," I called after her. "It's not a dog."

She stopped in her tracks and turned. "Then what is it?"

"What would you say if I told you I had gotten you on that Oprah show about Graduating Against the Odds?"

She just stood and looked at me, her mouth open.

"Well...?" I asked.

"What would I say? I cannot believe you, Robert Pardi Jr. You are the most amazing husband in the entire universe! How did you do it?"

"Baby, you know I would move mountains for you." I took her in my arms and held her close. It felt so good to make her so happy. "You are amazing," I whispered to her. "My God. Look at what you've accomplished. I am so proud of you."

"I can't believe you did this," Des repeated again and again. "Oprah!" She was over the moon.

I explained that I had already been in touch with her superiors at the hospital. They were happy to give her the time off and, with the help of her oncologist, I was also able to secure permission for the producers to film at the hospital.

When the producers interviewed her oncologist, he told them that Des was seriously ill, that the odds of the cancer returning were about 80 per cent and that she probably had only three years to live - the same prognosis he had given me some time before.

I nearly flew into a rage, but I contained myself. He had been a great and caring doctor, and I certainly I didn't want to jeopardize Des's appearance on Oprah, which I knew would mean so much to her. So I took the producers aside, explained that Des did not know this - if it were, in fact, true - and stipulated that the use of that interview was a deal-breaker. I have no idea how I would have explained the cancellation to Des but there was no way in hell that interview with that information was going to be broadcast.

When I explained to the lead producer the way Des had chosen to handle her cancer, not knowing the extent of her disease and having everything filtered through me, she listened quietly, and her stern, no-nonsense expression gave way to one of understanding. She got it, and I was beyond relieved.

She put her hand on my arm. "Not to worry, Mr. Pardi. We wish your wife a great career as a doctor with many, many more years of good health."

The segment was aired without the negative prognosis, and it was wonderful.

Oprah was at the height of her popularity then and it was a heady experience. They flew us out first class, put us up in a four-star hotel and transported us to the studio in a limo. In addition to filming at the hospital, they used photos of Des as a small child with her toy doctor's kit and a video tape of her graduation. They interviewed Des and she was able to tell her story...how she had entered the MD/PhD program thinking that she would go on to be a research scientist, but that her experience as a patient had changed that.

"Having gone through this would help me become even a better doctor than I might have been because now I had the patient's perspective, and that is an amazing, amazing thing to have. It was a gift handed to me, essentially."

She also talked about how, at one point, she really thought she was going to die, but she kept going. The camera panned to the audience and the women were teary-eyed.

Then, after they showed the tape, Oprah, with a big smile on her face, turned to a radiant Des coming out from behind a curtain and said, "Please welcome Dr. Desiree Pardi!"

Des had the biggest smile on her face that I had ever seen. The audience responded with huge applause and Des. Oprah stood with her arms open and in a rush of enthusiasm, Des dove right in and gave Oprah a huge hug.

"No honorary doctor here," Oprah said, alluding to her own, recently awarded, honorary PhD. "You earned every single moment of it, every single step of the fight you did."

Des went on to mention our relationship and how my love had given her strength. Oprah liked that and threw some of the focus to me.

"Everybody wants a partner like Robert...Everybody wants somebody who thinks you're beautiful when you're bald, beautiful no matter what."

The camera panned to me. There I was sitting in the audience with tears in my eyes for millions of viewers to see. But that was OK. I looked at my wife and saw a miracle: Dr. Desiree Pardi, MD and PhD. She had done it. Her latest tests were good. She looked healthy and beyond happy. At that point she had, indeed, beaten the odds.

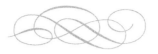

Chapter 21

As part of her internship, Des saw many cancer patients, and it became clear early on that she was especially good at caring for them. It was not just her rock-solid knowledge, it was, of course, the experience of having had cancer - an experience that informed how she handled patients, but one that she never shared with them. That experience, and the honest, direct, yet totally comforting manner in which she interacted with patients, made her a superior physician from the get-go. She had compassion. She had walked in their shoes and she knew how difficult it could be, how frightening, how alienating. She treated her patients like people, not just notations on a hospital chart. She was practicing palliative care without putting a name to it.

Des was thriving...or so it would seem. In February, 2003, however, her doctor gave me some entirely unexpected and upsetting news: her cancer markers - the blood test results that indicate active malignancy - were up and her most recent CT scan revealed that the cancer had metastasized to her liver with two lesions.

I was incredulous. She had been doing so well. I was overwhelmed with a sense of dread.

Des, on the other hand, was almost relieved. "I've been living with this Sword of Damocles over my head for too long," she said, fighting back tears. "Now I'm relieved. I don't have to wait for it to happen. I knew it was possible and probable."

I didn't cry, but I sure as hell wanted to. Des hadn't talked about that feeling of foreboding since her depression, a few years before. She never shared she thought it was "possible and probable". It must have been awful walking around with that fear, and I was angry with myself for somehow not knowing.

I fell back into an earlier pattern and began drinking to cope. I had never wanted it to get out of hand because I didn't want, in any way, to be like my father. But at that point, I found myself sneaking drinks, bringing back wine in paper cups from the pizza place, or taking walks with a "coffee cup" in hand. I never expected the cancer to return. I had been blind-sided, better yet sucker-punched.

I hated myself for adding drinking to our mix, but I found it was the only way I could cope. Somewhere deep inside I felt like I failed and like everything was ending. Des coped by not wanting to know every last detail of her disease. I coped by anesthetizing myself. Des told friends that she was worried about me. She said that it hurt her unbearably to see me so sad and defeated. With all this woman continued to go through, she was worried about me!

It tore my guts out to watch her going through chemotherapy yet again, and one night, while we were visiting my mother, it all got the better of me. I was having yet another drink and my mother started harping on me.

"You've become just like your father," she yelled. "Exactly like him!"

That did it. It was the proverbial straw.

"Do you have any idea what is happening in my life, do you?" I screamed at her. "No, you don't. You don't know how it feels. I can't save her. Don't you get it? I can't save Desiree! I should just kill myself," I screamed back, tears of rage and pain clouding my vision. I grabbed a kitchen knife. I was spiraling. I swear the only thing that prevented me from plunging it in was the look on Des's face. As miserable as I felt, and as much as the pain and hurt were tearing me apart, I saw the look of concern on her face for me. This is not the way it should be. She had asked me to be her rock.

What the fuck are you doing Robert?, I thought to myself.

The empathetic, compassionate look on her face and that questioning voice booming in my mind shocked me back to reality. I needed to learn to surrender and let go of what I couldn't control. I needed to stop fighting against life and trying to save her. I needed to start fighting for our life together, regardless of the remaining time we had left. It all became clear in an instant. I collapsed on the floor. Des came over to me, hugged me from behind as she always had, pressing her body into me, letting me know we were one and whispered, "I love you Robert Pardi. It is all going to be ok."

I never drank to excess again after that. I realized that the numbing was preventing me from feeling what I needed to feel on my skin. I needed to let go of my ego, drop my shield of alcohol and live what she, what I, what we were going through to be able to manage it in the best way possible. Hiding only made me weaker.

We quickly got back on a normal footing - normal, that is, for a couple living with the cancer that had so invaded our lives. Des continued to endure all her treatments with a smile, fitting it into her schedule as though it were just some appointment she had to keep once a week, arranging it for a time when she could have the following day to recuperate. It never interfered with her rounds at the hospital. Ever. She was totally motivated to do her job tending to patients. It was all she focused on. Amazing when I look back at it. And I was back to being her defender, her advocate, her shield and it filled me with such purpose that it actually became a lighter burden to carry than I could have imagined.

On one of her days off, we went to the Hamptons and took a walk on the beach. Ever since the beginning of our relationship, the beach had been an important part of our lives together. We both loved smelling the fresh, salty air and feeling the sand between our toes and beneath our feet. Over the years, we had gone to Florida, Puerto Rico, and the Caribbean many, many times, traveling as frequently as once a month. These jaunts ate up an awful lot of money and kept me constantly behind the eight ball, but they were important because they helped keep Des's spirits up.

My relationship with money had never been good. We had always spent way too much of it, and when Des got sick, money totally lost any significance. Thank God for credit cards! Des loved the beach and that was that - whatever it took.

On this particular day in the Hamptons, we walked silently, just holding hands, enjoying sand, the lapping water and the sunset, but then Des turned to me and with the sweetest look on her face said, "Robert, please stop worrying. I'm feeling fine...I'll be fine. Really. Maybe it will not go away, maybe this will be a chronic disease I, we, will need to live around but please stop worrying."

She then squeezed my hand, that amazing, loving form of communication that was asking me to stay present and not lose myself in future focused fears.

I must have seemed worried, and I wanted to smack myself. I never wanted her to see that again. "Of course you will be," I said, trying to convince myself...trying not to think about what the doctor had said about Des having an 80 per cent chance of her cancer recurring and that she would most likely be dead in three years. *New drugs are coming out all the time*, I forced myself to think, but I couldn't actually say to her because that would be verbalizing what I was so afraid of – that despite her endless optimism and all our precautions, she knew deep inside, how really dire her situation was.

Des smiled and said, "Come on...I'll race you to the water." She dropped my hand and took off. I followed, caught up with her, grabbed her and held her close. Neither of us spoke a word as we both stepped onto the wet sand and pressed our feet in, side by side.

I looked down and saw the impressions of our feet. I pulled the camera from my pocket and snapped some photos. We had always taken pictures when we made impressions in the sand and had dozens, if not hundreds, in a big box in our closet. I couldn't help but to wonder how many more trips and how many more photos we would get to take after that.

At this point, Des had finished her internship and had moved into her residency in Internal Medicine and was putting in some pretty heavy hours. I don't know how she did it. It was tough for even those with no medical problems, but Des was unstoppable, and she was blossoming as a physician. Her enthusiasm for her work was unbridled and her patients loved her - especially the cancer patients. First and foremost, she allowed them their dignity, and that was something so many of them had been robbed of in the course of their treatments. She gave them great care and showed deep compassion, and perhaps some of them sensed that "Dr. Des" had an extra reason for being able to understand all the things they were able to communicate - and all the things they weren't.

Des had worked so hard to get to this place and I loved seeing her come through the door of our apartment, at the end of her shift, looking so damned cute in her white doctor's coat, tired but fulfilled from her day. Unfortunately, I was not able to say the same about my own day. My work, as limited as it had become, had ceased to be any kind of focus for me, and I found myself looking for reasons not to travel back to Dubai on the schedule I had created. I spent most of my time pouring over cancer statistics and articles that I could almost understand. There had to be something that would stop this thing from taking over Des's body. *Something.*

Des was all I was focused on. I began packing her lunches to make sure she was getting the right nutrition: high fiber and high protein foods like nuts and seeds, Greek yoghurt, lots of salads, grains and fresh vegetables. I walked the couple of blocks to work with her every morning and called for her at the end of the day. I felt compelled to, or else something terrible would happen. It was almost like not stepping on the cracks in the sidewalk.

The chemotherapy took care of one of the lesions, but the second one was resistant. There was just so much chemo her body could take, so her oncologist suggested that they go in for it surgically.

"I know you don't want to hear the specifics, Des," I said to her, "but Dr. Samuels is thinking of doing something a bit radical which would involve surgery."

Des just looked at me with a sweet smile. "You're empowered to make all my decisions."

"I would feel more comfortable getting your input. I am pretty sure I know the answer, but I need your guidance," I said.

"Well, if we're talking about a choice between more chemo and surgery," Des responded, "I'll choose the surgery."

I expected that surgery would be her choice, because she always opted for the most aggressive treatment. So the decision was made and Des went into the hospital for a liver resection, a procedure where the cancerous part of the liver is removed. The pain was severe and the epidural - a regional anesthesia that blocks pain - had fallen out. We called for a nurse. No one came. I called again. Nothing. It was a nightmare.

I couldn't believe it. Forget that Des was a doctor, a comrade in arms. Here was a stage 4 cancer patient - the staging had recently been upped from 3 to metastatic - who had just had major surgery and they were allowing her to lie there in agony. It destroyed me to see her in pain like that, and the anger bubbled up. I went down the hall and the nurses were all laughing and gabbing and paying absolutely no attention to what they were supposed to be doing - looking after patients.

I raised my voice, told them what was going on and all they had to say was "be patient." Be patient, my ass! What was wrong with these people? My wife is lying there in agony while they were laughing and gossiping, and they want me to be patient! Had they totally lost sight of people? Of a person's dignity? How could they just leave someone writhing in pain? They didn't deserve to be called nurses.

I had enough and it was time to play the Ace in my pocket. I had the cell phone number of the Chief Resident, who Des knew, and the pain meds were taken care of instantly. Somewhere during that incident, Des had specifically asked for the heavy-duty painkiller Dilaudid, because she knew it would help alleviate the extreme pain she was experiencing. Well, the fact that she had specifically requested Dilaudid was noted on her record and that labeled her as a "drug seeker." If the whole episode hadn't been so horrible, it would almost have been laughable - a cancer patient who was knowledgeable because she herself was a physician asking for relief of unbearable pain being called a "drug seeker."

We are more caring of animals. They allowed a patient to lie there in agony and then add insult to injury by labeling her a "drug seeker. Had any of them had part of their liver removed? I really had to contain my rage. It was unconscionable.

Des, with her amazing can-do attitude, recouped and was soon back at the hospital taking care of patients as though she were the healthiest person on the premises. I, on the other hand, fought to not spiral into the black hole of despair. With all the research I was doing and with all the inquiries I was making, I was coming up with zero. I wanted to have a back-up plan, just in case. Yet, there were no efficacious new drugs available, and I was terrified of losing her. I had cut my trips to Dubai to once every six months and, for all practical purposes, was uninvolved in my business. The demands of managing Desiree's care as well as looking after her consumed more and more of my time and just about all of my mental energy. I could think of little else. I was fortunate that my friend and business partner Khaled gave me all the time I needed to pursue, as he so graciously put it, "a much bigger job is calling for you now my brother, caring for the woman you love."

Slowly I let go of the dream of succeeding in finance. I think I had always known that I would have to lose in order for Desiree to win, but I accepted it fully and joyfully and with tremendous gratitude to my friend who gave me all the room I needed to keep Des going. His level of understanding is something I still marvel at, to this day. We have remained good friends, and I will always be grateful to him. Always.

Des knew how upset I was. There was no way to keep it from her and she blamed herself.

"Look what I've done to your business, your life," she said shaking her head, her eyes welling with tears. "I am so sorry, Robert, so, so sorry. Can you ever forgive me?"

"Forgive you? Baby, I love you. You are my life - the most important thing on God's earth to me." I wrapped my arms around her. "If there were any way I could take the cancer for you, I would. Baby, it is a job, a job, you are my purpose – that trumps a job any day, ok?"

Then she cried, letting loose so many months, if not years, of pent-up tears. "And I cried as well. There was no way I couldn't. We held on to each other, just sobbing. We had both kept it pent up for so long, we had to let it out. We kept on crying and holding on to each other until we had no tears left. And then we started laughing - loud, uncontrollable laughs, like a couple of goofy kids. It always amazed me, regardless of how difficult or dark things seemed to be, she and I had the ability to laugh, wholeheartedly.

"I'm hungry," Des announced, in the middle of shrieks of laughter.

"So am I!" I answered, practically snorting my words.

So we washed our faces, left the apartment and went to our favorite Italian restaurant for some good veal and peppers. We insisted on a booth so that we could sit side by side with our bodies touching one another.

When we got home we made love so slowly, never wanting to stop...never wanting to let go of one another for even a brief moment, let alone for all of eternity.

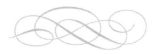

Chapter 22

Des was deeply affected by that incident in the hospital. "That is hardly the way to treat patients!" she said over and over. "I would never let a patient of mine lie there in such pain. It is absolutely cruel. And what about having some respect for the patient? Their dignity? Patients are people, human beings, not just some faceless creatures lying in hospital beds with numbers on charts hanging off the ends of those beds. This kind of treatment is unconscionable and it's the kind of thing I absolutely can do something about...something I <u>will</u> do something about."

She was coming closer and closer to formally changing her area of concentration. Palliative Care as a discipline was relatively new then. Born out of the hospice movement, which in itself, had only really existed in the U.S. since the early 80's, palliative care is about treating the whole patient and meeting his or her overall needs as an individual...and really taking into consideration the patient's goals. While not limited to hospice patients, who are terminal with six or fewer months to live, palliative care health professionals and doctors treat any patient who is dealing with a chronic or serious illness, often from the onset of the illness. The administration of pain medication is certainly a huge part of palliative care, but it goes way beyond that. As my friend Claire Altman, the former Chief Operating Officer of the HealthCare Chaplaincy in New York explains, "Palliative Care improves the quality of life of patients with a serious or chronic illness as well as their families, matches treatment to the patient's values and goals, relieves suffering, and treats the whole person - body, mind, and spirit."

Dr. Diane Meier, founder and former Director of the Center to Advance Palliative Care and Vice-Chair for Public Policy, as well as distinguished Professor of Geriatrics and Palliative Medicine and Catherine Gaisman Professor of Medical Ethics at the Icahn School of Medicine at Mount Sinai, and now Director Emerita and Medical Advisor to CAPC, explain that palliative care is a team approach.

"The team spends as much time as necessary with you and your family. They become a partner with you and your other doctors. They support you and your family every step of the way, not only by controlling your symptoms, but also by helping you to understand your treatment options and how they will help you achieve your goals."

A palliative care team is usually made up of medical, nursing and allied health professionals who offer a range of services to assist the patient, family and caregivers throughout the arch of illness.

According to the *New York Times,* today Palliative Care is one of the fastest-growing fields in medicine. At the time, it clearly wasn't and Des knew from personal experience what a void in the system there was. She talked more and more about it.

At this point, she was in her final year of residency in Internal Medicine and tests revealed that even after all the chemo that she endured, as well as the liver resection, there was further metastasis. It became harder and harder for us both to stick with her original resolution of not wanting to know all the specifics, but we did. I had also learned to not let anything show on my face and it also meant that I needed to stop talking to anyone about what was going on because I could not control what might show on their face. So I made the decision to go at it alone from that point forward.

All Des knew was that she needed yet more chemo. I knew she was in very real trouble. Her oncologist had said that when he talked to the Oprah producer the day of filming. I couldn't allow myself to really hear it, to really think it, but now the doctor was telling me more directly: we had come to a point in time where

Desiree was unlikely to survive and most likely had only a short time left to live.

My whole body went numb and I was unable to speak. On some level I may have known this, but I didn't want to hear it. I didn't want that death sentence to be formalized in words. And as much as we valued the great care this wonderful doctor had given her for some time, and the esteem in which both Des and I held him, I couldn't accept it. I felt we could do more – that we had to do more. There had to be other options out there – no matter how difficult to tolerate, because that's what Des would want. She always chose the most aggressive options.

As I was leaving, one of the nurses in the area who was very close to Des noticed how distraught I was and she took me aside.

"I know I shouldn't say this to you, Rob, but there's a doctor I've heard incredible things about. He does things a lot differently. He thinks out of the box and he's amazing. He has saved many, many lives."

She had my attention.

"His name is Mitchell Gaynor. You should go see him."

She quickly wrote down the name and number for me. I had never heard of this doctor, but I wasn't about to let any lead go uninvestigated, especially when I heard the words "he saves lives."

I asked around and did my homework and I learned that this Dr. Gaynor, a hematologist and oncologist, had a formidable background. He had been at the Rockefeller Institute and Strang Cancer Prevention Clinic and had written a few books. Plus he had tons of patients - cancer survivors - who adored him. The many, many survivors who he cared for attested to the efficacy of his using complementary therapies in addition to orthodox cancer treatments.

I definitely wanted her to consult with this doctor, but I was unsure how I was going to approach Des with the idea, because I did not want to undermine her faith in Dr. Samuels, who so knowledgeably and compassionately had shepherded her to this point. We both thought the world of him.

"No way!" Des said when I suggested it. "That guy is off the charts."

I wanted to say..."but he saves lives," but I stopped myself. That would mean that hers was in imminent danger - and that information was not on the table.

"Ah, come on, Des. I heard he's very good. He studied at Rockefeller, headed up Strang, and he's an assistant professor at Weill. He can't be all that weird," I said.

"Yeah, but I heard he's into meditating and chanting. I hate that stuff. It's not science. It's all a goddamned waste of time. Do you really think some herbs and incents are going to make a difference?"

We were at the end of the line. I had to convince her. "Come on, Baby," I said, putting my arms around her. "Let's go see for ourselves. I know you like to take the most aggressive approach to things and sometimes aggressive means radical as well."

"I wouldn't quite consider herbs and meditating either radical or aggressive," Des said. "More like crazy."

"What do we have to lose?" I asked. "I've read that herbal treatments are gaining some acceptance. Sometimes aggressive also means thinking outside the box, right?"

She didn't answer.

"Come on, do it for me," I pleaded.

But Des insisted she was not interested - and while I didn't want to scare her, I was desperate. So I kept at her, and didn't stop.

"I'm part of this too, you know, and I really, really need you to do this. I want you to have every tool at your disposal."

"Gee-sus! All right," Des said, totally exasperated. "If it's that important to you, I'll go!" Then she stomped off into the other room.

No matter. She would go! Thank God.

When I called to make the appointment, I was told there was a three-month wait. We didn't have three months to wait, so I explained that Des was a physician. Could they extend professional courtesy? I held my breath thinking how odd it was that I never knew such a thing even existed a few years ago. Yes they could. They found a slot for us, and we were given an appointment for the following week.

A day or so later, I gathered Des's records and took them to Dr. Gaynor's office. In addition to wanting to drop the records off, I needed to explain our way of doing things...Des's coping mechanism, her not wanting to know all the details of her malignancies, our need for all the information to be funneled through me. For the first time in all the years that Des had been sick, and all the doctors and nurses she had seen, no eyebrows were raised, and no one looked at me like I had two heads.

"No problem, Mr. Pardi," the sweet woman at the desk said. "We'll brief the doctor."

I knew, at that moment, this was the oncology office for us. It just felt good.

We arrived for the appointment but Des was beyond skeptical. Dr. Gaynor's office was on the ground floor of an old townhouse and nothing about it looked like a physician's office. There were plants and flowers all around and large, color photographs of Hindu temples and East Asian Indians in colorful dress. Tea was brewing in the corner and the air smelled of spices. Gentle chanting wafted from a sound system. Phones were ringing, messengers were coming in and out, and we could hear rolling laughter coming from a room in the back.

I must have looked surprised to hear that because one of the two women at the desk said matter-of-factly, "Oh, that's some of our patients. They're having chemo." Both women smiled then went on with their work. Joyful laughter in the chemo room? Nothing about the place said "cancer."

The doctor came out to greet us. He was fiftyish, average height with a handsome, boyish face and dark curly hair. When he smiled, it was a wonderful, warm open smile that said this is a doctor who cares, and when he reached out to greet us, I could see Des relax, ever so slightly. She quickly went on to say, however, "I'm here because my husband wanted me to come."

That didn't seem to faze Dr. Gaynor at all. He smiled, ushered us into his office, asked us to make ourselves comfortable and, for more than two hours, he was oncologist, medical colleague, shrink, and spiritual guide. Both Des and I had been raised as Roman Catholics and while neither of us were religious, we did have ingrained beliefs. Dr. Gaynor's beliefs, which informed his worldviews and his approaches to life and healing, were light years from ours. He believed in Karma and what he called "The Divine" and it was all strange and surprising - especially coming from a Westerner. But he was smart and soothing, and I could see he was getting through to Des just a little bit.

"I've been pretty sick," she said, "and lately I've been thinking I'm going to die." She paused and looked at him. "Am I going to die?" she asked, quite directly.

Am I going to die? My heart sank at hearing Des ask that. She had never expressed that fear to me, even though she must have been living with it for a very long time. I was also terrified that he would tell her that she probably had only a couple of years left, at best, and I was just about to say something - anything - to stop that from happening when Dr. Gaynor said something I was not at all expecting.

"Yes, of course, at some point," he said gently, "just as I am and your husband is and everyone we care about, for that matter. But none of us knows when." He paused, then looked at us both. "We are here today, and every day of our human birth is a gift from The Divine. It's our mission to live each day with joy and to bring happiness to ourselves, as well as others."

I was beyond relieved and grateful. His words were soothing, and I hoped Des was feeling that. She just sat and listened quietly.

"What do you want most, this very moment?" Dr. Gaynor asked her.

"I want more energy," Des was quick to answer. "I need more energy to work."

He smiled at that. "And what do you <u>really</u> want?"

Des didn't have to think to answer that. "I want to live life as best I can."

"And you will," Dr. Gaynor said, leaning forward. "But above all, you must learn to love yourself. That's the most healing thing of all."

Des glanced at me, then she squeezed my hand and I knew she was easing into accepting this doctor who was unlike any we had ever encountered - and we had certainly encountered many in the past few years.

Dr. Gaynor then asked me to leave and wait in the other room. Aside from that gynecologist appointment several years prior, I had never left Des alone during an examination, and I had never been asked to leave before either. But there was something about the man that made me feel confident. Then Des squeezed my hand again - always our "silent signal," and I had no problem respecting his request.

While he was examining Des and taking blood for his own tests, I went out to the waiting room, where I was able to have a close look at the photographs the doctor had on the walls. When I asked the receptionist about the Hindu temple and the people in traditional garb, she explained that the doctor was a committed supporter of an Indian holy man named Amma, and that he traveled there frequently and helped Amma build a much-needed hospital in a very poor area of India.

I must admit, on top of his superior academic and medical credentials, this was just one more reason Dr. Gaynor was such an unusual physician. And when he had me rejoin him and Des after her exam, I felt even more positive about our having gone to him.

He told us that he agreed with the current chemo regimen Dr. Samuels had put Des on and then proceeded to go through his protocol of herbs and vitamins designed to help boost energy and the body's immune system...herbs such as Tumeric, Ashwaganda, and Genistein...vitamins such as C, and D3...amino acids, L Glutamine and mushrooms, especially the extract Maitake D. He also recommended several cups a day of green tea and cautioned about sugar, which he said was a negative for everyone but especially for cancer patients, because it feeds the cancer cells. I had never heard that one before.

Then he urged Des to come to his next meditation session. Meditation, he explained, was key to stress reduction and healthy living. Des and I looked at each other. That was a stretch, since neither one of us had ever sat still for more than two minutes at a time in our entire lives.

We said our goodbyes and as we were leaving the office Des laughed. "Meditation! Right. Just what I want to do with my time."

I had to agree with her, but I didn't want the idea of meditation to put the kibosh on the whole thing.

"Forget the meditation for a moment. Aside from that, what do you think?" I asked her.

"I think that he's a really nice man and he does have amazing credentials. And he did make a very good argument for supplement use, because I do agree that there might be something to be said for the way some supplements and herbs could be used to help protect the good cells and also help bolster T cells. I just don't know about all that other stuff. Do you know that after he examined me, he played some kind of sound machine and placed the speaker on what he said was my 'heart chakra' so that the sound could penetrate? It was some kind of chanting. Sound penetration? Chanting? What the kind of medicine is that?"

My heart sank. She wasn't going to go for it.

"But, I have to say, Robert, that I really did like that chanting!"

Well, Well, that's a start, I thought. *Now if I can only convince her to continue with him…*

At home, later that day, Des put on the chanting CD Dr. Gaynor had given her and I watched with relief as she listened to it. Headphones on, her eyes gently closed, she seemed so peaceful, and I was already grateful to the doctor.

I badgered her and was able to convince her to go to the big meditation session Dr. Gaynor had suggested. It took place in a very large living room of an apartment on Central Park West, the home of one of his patients, who we later learned was, at that point, an eight-year survivor of stage 4 pancreatic cancer - the cancer that nearly always kills within months of diagnosis. We watched while a room full of people, most of them his patients, we assumed, listened to him talk about negative and positive energy and how aligning yourself with the positives can change your life... and how grateful we should be for every day and how we should look for the joy in that day.

We watched how everyone eagerly closed their eyes and went into a deep state of relaxation as the doctor played a Tibetan bowl - a large, shiny brass bowl that he struck with a felt-covered hammer while he chanted a rhythmic, soothing prayer. We saw the serene looks on their faces and how happy and peaceful they looked as they left to go home. I wasn't quite into it, and kept opening my eyes, but that didn't matter a bit because I saw the serene look on Des's face and that was all I cared about.

Each time we went, Des got more and more into the whole program. I was still a voyeur, too invested in the outcome to relax and get into anything, but as I watched her gain strength, I was cautiously optimistic. While we continued with Des's primary on-cologist, we started regular visits to Dr. Gaynor for his support and complementary therapies. He sent Des to an acupuncturist, prescribed green drink mixes, gave her additional CDs so that she could do her own sound therapy and reviewed daily meditations with her. He also pressed her to eat only organic food, juice regularly with carrots, watercress, green apples, ginger and beets, and continue with the daily regimen of supplements.

The job of ordering the dozens of supplements, dividing them up into the several doses needed throughout the day and making sure Des took them fell to me, as did the juicing preparation and making sure she ate properly. Sometimes Des would give me a hard time, like when she was in a rush to get to the hospital to see patients, and I would harangue her - but she always gave in because she was looking so good and feeling so good. All of Dr. Gaynor's extras had to be the reason.

She was still doing monthly chemotherapy, which she took with her regular oncologist, but as the weeks went by and she became more and more invested in Dr. Gaynor's approach, she was thinking of making a change.

"I'm thinking seriously of moving all my care to Dr. Gaynor," she said one night after a particularly long day at work. "I prefer the privacy here...I really don't like running into colleagues at the hospital when I'm on my way for treatments and besides, here it is almost 8 o'clock at night, I've been on my feet all day at the hospital, and I'm still full of energy. Dr. Gaynor's really on to something."

And thank God for that. I couldn't believe it. My heart filled when I looked at her. She hadn't looked that good in at least three years.

She caught me staring.

"What?"

"Just looking at my beautiful wife."

"I'm only looking good because you take such good care of me - even if sometimes you really piss me off!"

It was hard when she got angry with me, but I definitely was taking good care of her and it was all that mattered to me. Everything else in my life - friends, family and work - seemed to have faded away. I was on kind of a suspended animation with my job. I did the barest minimum to stay connected to the company. Khaled continued to be supportive and while he did cut my salary back, some money was still coming in, and with the modest money that Desiree was now earning, we were able to make it.

"Come on, Baby," I said. "Let's get some rest. Chemo tomorrow."

We were due at the hospital first thing the next morning, but Des had made other arrangements. Aside from her discomfort with running into her fellow interns and others she worked with and the way she felt it compromised her dignity, she was getting to know Dr. Gaynor as a colleague as well as her own physician and the man that she had originally dismissed as "off the wall," she had come to regard as the smartest doctor she had ever met.

"It's time to make that change we've been talking about," she said looking at me a bit impishly. "Well, actually I've gone ahead and done it. We'll be going to Gaynor's for chemo."

She thought I might have been upset because she went ahead and did it without my final stamp of approval, but I couldn't have been happier. This showed me that she felt empowered, and that was so important going forward. And while we both liked and admired Dr. Samuels greatly, and were so appreciative of all he had done for Des, over the weeks she had been going to Dr. Gaynor I had come to believe that he was her only chance for survival.

"He knows how to treat the whole patient, and it's so much better at his office," Des said. "I have my dignity there and besides, where else can you hear laughter coming from a chemotherapy room?"

She smiled at me, and I smiled back. I finally had reason to hope.

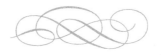

Chapter 23

So now we were 100 per cent on board with Dr. Gaynor...the supplements, the healthful organic food, juicing with fresh vegetables, meditations, sound therapy - even changing to a mattress made of organic materials, because Dr. Gaynor had advised us to cut out as much toxicity from our environment as we could. Following all his guidelines was a lot of work, but Des was doing great, and that was the bottom line. Her markers were good, and she was able to stop the chemo.

The next time we were in his office, Dr. Gaynor suggested we come to a puja. "I think you'll like it," he said, with a big smile. "There's chanting."

I had no idea what a puja was, but I knew that Des really enjoyed listening to the chanting disks Dr. Gaynor had given her.

"There's something so peaceful about it," she explained to me. "I have no idea what they're saying, of course. It's in Hindi, but on a visceral level, I understand every word."

She did look incredibly peaceful while she was listening to chanting. Sometimes I used to just sit and stare at her while she was curled up on the chair in the corner, big headphones like giant muffs on her ears. Chanting wasn't something I cared to do myself, but I sure liked what it did for Des.

"So what's a puja?" I asked the doctor.

"Why don't you just come and see? It's Monday night at my apartment," he said as he scribbled his address on a piece of paper and handed it to me. "Hope you can make it."

"If there's chanting," Des said, with that childlike wonder that filled her voice whenever she was discovering something new, "I want to go."

So we went, of course, and that evening proved to be the beginning of a completely new phase of our lives.

When we arrived at Dr. Gaynor's Central Park West apartment, we were greeted by several pairs of shoes right outside his door. We quickly learned that shoes were off limits in the Gaynor home. Aside from showing respect for The Divine, we would later learn, there was also a very practical reason: why bring the muck and grime of the New York City streets into the sanctity of one's home?

"Duh!" Des said shaking her head. "Never learned *that* in med school and it's so obvious. No more shoes in our house!" she laughed. I laughed, too, because it was kind of obvious.

There were lots of people inside the apartment...several seated in the spacious and beautifully decorated living room...some on the sofa and chairs, some crossed-legged on the floor...some old, some young, and all in a mix of races and nationalities. While we didn't know their names, we recognized several of Dr. Gaynor's patients and smiled "hello." Some people were quietly engaged in discussion. Others were sitting in silent contemplation, their focus on the large portrait of Amma that was set on the floor in an elaborate makeshift altar near the far end of the room.

It all seemed totally out of context with the spare, modern furnishings and contemporary sculptures and artwork in the apartment. A benevolent-looking young Indian man, whose photograph we had seen in the doctor's office, bare chested and in traditional Indian garb, looked out at us with an intense gaze from the large, golden framed painting. The frame was draped with a garland of flowers, and all around were tiny Hindu statues and bouquets of red and peach roses and deep pink peonies. Amma, we had learned, while in the body of a man, was female incarnate. It was a hard concept for us to grasp, initially, but we learned to appreciate it, if not fully understand it.

"Good to see you both!" Dr. Gaynor said, greeting us with his warm, wide smile as he came by from another room. "Get yourselves settled in. We'll be starting soon."

The chairs were all taken so we found a spot on the floor. I sat first, then Des nestled up against me.

Soon the doctor began. Sri Naranyni Amma, he explained, the young man in the painting, was an incarnation of The Divine who was sent to earth during *Kali Yuga*, especially negative and difficult times, such as those we were experiencing. These puja prayer sessions, he continued, were to honor and connect with him.

I think my whole body must have stiffened then, because Des turned and whispered, "What's wrong?"

"What's wrong? Supplements and meditation were one thing - but this?" raced through my head.

I was so afraid this was way too radical, and it would destroy all the work I put into convincing her to move her care to him.

But before I even had the chance to response, the doctor started chanting. There was something so calming, so hypnotic about it. I had no idea what he was saying, but I just squeezed Des's shoulder and ever so slightly, let myself go with it.

Des, on the other hand, really went with it and I felt her body totally relax as she hummed along. She even knew some of the words and would include them whenever she could.

The chanting continued for about an hour and the entire time Des was totally peaceful and still. After the chanting, some of the water that Dr. Gaynor had sanctified during the ceremony was passed around in small cups. We watched as everyone drank from their cups and then sprinkled themselves with the remaining drops.

Des and I looked at each other. "Hey, when in Rome..." I said as I drank the water and then patted my forehead and hair. Des did the same and it all seemed perfectly natural and normal. I had to laugh to myself. I hadn't been to the holy water font in church in years, and here I was anointing myself out of a paper cup as part of a Hindu rite.

But both of us sat out the next part. One by one, everyone got up, went to the altar, got down on their hands and knees and paid deference to Amma. Using their hands to sweep it towards their faces, they inhaled the smoke that was coming from a small oil lamp. Then they picked up several rose petals that were scattered about and tossed them around the base of the painting. When they got up to make way for the next person, everyone seemed blessed and so serene - kind of like when we take communion. I wondered if they had to go to some kind of confession beforehand.

After all of that, the rest of the evening was fun. Everyone had been asked to bring a vegetarian dish for a potluck dinner. The food was varied and plentiful and the talk and socializing was easy, with lots of laughter and friendly chatter. We met a couple of physicians, an architect, some artists, a psychologist, an importer, and many totally western Amma devotees who had made pilgrimages to his ashram, an enclave in Southern India based around his religious temple.

We had no way of knowing, that night, what close, personal friends we would become with both Mitch Gaynor and his then wife Cathy, nor how meaningful Amma would be to us and how his mission to serve those who were poor and in ill health would impact our lives.

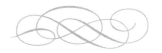

Chapter 24

When Des graduated from her residency program at New York Presbyterian Hospital/Weil Cornell, in June 2005, it was a great day. She had soldiered on and climbed yet another ladder in her medical training. And to make the event even more special, that night, at the festivities that were held in the grand ballroom of New York's Roosevelt Hotel, she was presented with "The Compassionate Care Award," an honor given to a doctor who "exemplifies warmth, compassion and human decency in caring for patients. The award was the legacy of a patient who had received such compassionate care that she wanted the physician who delivered that care to be recognized. Des's award was presented to her by Dr. Mark Pecker, a doctor to whom she had become very close and who clearly marveled, as did I, at Des's strength and sense of purpose, despite everything she continued to battle. Her ability to care for patients in the most compassionate way was clear to all of her colleagues, many of whom, by now, were aware of her personal struggle. She got a standing ovation and my heart swelled with pride. My girl was amazing. The evening was made even more special because the students had chosen to honor Dr. Pecker for his exceptional abilities as a teacher and they selected Desiree to present the award. She glowed as both giver and receiver and it was an unforgettable, beyond special evening.

For a moment, I allowed myself to forget all that we had been through to get her to this point, basking in the reflective light...the proud husband of an extraordinary woman for whom my love and admiration grew more and more as every day went by.

The palliative care sensibility that had come to define Des was clearly front and center, so it came as no surprise to anyone when she went on to become a Fellow in the Department of Neurology, Division of Pain and Palliative Medicine, at Memorial Sloan Kettering, one of the world's premier cancer centers.

Des was clearly in the right place and she was ebullient and while by now many of her colleagues knew that she had breast cancer, she rarely talked about it. There were times, however, that her schedule had to be adjusted for medical appointments of her own. I remember the other fellows and residents being in awe of how she handled her situation. She was in the hardest fight of her life but had chosen to make it just a part of her life. To Des, her own cancer - as tough as it was - was just something she had to take care of, and not what got her up in the morning, drove her through often exhausting days and brought her home at night still filled with the struggles of patients she had encountered and things she could do to help ease their journeys.

I marveled at her, myself. I knew she was a strong woman, but the depth of her strength was almost otherworldly. For me, knowing the extent of her cancer and the statistics that informed the diagnosis, it was a constant struggle to be up and positive and never let her see how frightened I really was.

At this point, Des had to undergo yet another round of chemotherapy. This time the drug didn't cause her to lose her hair, and she was grateful. Her hair had grown back in and she had gone back to her trademark long, blonde hair, which made her happy.

"I'm so glad I don't have to wear a wig," she said with a big smile. "I just love the way it feels when the breeze goes through my hair when we take a ride and I keep the windows down." My girl always found the positive in just about every situation and even though I had just ordered her six new wigs, I was more than happy to relegate them to the back of the closet.

By this time, Des and Mitch Gaynor had become close, working colleagues, always eager to exchange ideas about the most effective ways of dealing with disease, and dealing with it in ways that could be most meaningful for their patients. Des and I were impressed with the steady stream of cancer patients Dr. Gaynor seemed to pluck from death's doorstep, including many other women with breast cancer. He was an extremely gifted doctor, and I will always be grateful to that hospital nurse who pulled me aside and whispered his name in my ear.

Des's and Dr. Gaynor's patient-doctor relationship had progressed to a professional doctor-doctor collaboration and soon it transitioned to a warm friendship for the four of us. We often spent weekends at the Gaynors' wonderful old Victorian house in Columbia County, at the foot of the Berkshires. The area is rich in history and Cathy and Des loved to tour the area and see the many churches, cemeteries and 18th and 19th century houses in the area. Both voracious readers and lovers of history, they always had tons to talk about.

Des had always been interested in the underground railway, the network of right-minded, courageous people who provided shelter for slaves escaping the pre-Civil War south. I think it was her really strong sense of fair-mindedness and justice that prompted this interest. One of her favorite books was Professor Henry Louis Gates's "The Classic Slave Narratives." She also liked reading about adventuresome women and she and Cathy could spend hours discussing books they had both read. Beryl Markam's "West with the Night," about a female pilot who lived in East Africa and Lillian Schlissel's "Women's Diaries of the Westward Journey" about the difficult trek westward made by more than 200,000 people in the mid-19th century were favorites. This is not to say, by the way, that Des didn't indulge in less lofty reads. She still loved spy novels, the "Shopaholic" series and an occasional "bodice ripper," just for fun. It was so "Des" to have such divergent interests - and to be enthusiastic about them all.

While Des and Cathy were out exploring, Mitch, the Gaynors' two young sons and I spent time with the four Scottish Long Horns the Gaynors had adopted. They had actually adopted three: two steers and a heifer. They had no idea that the female was pregnant and not long after, there were four! The adoptions came out of Mitch's Hindu sensibility and for me, strictly a city kid, it was fun, as were our trips to the local farm equipment store and the parks.

Sometimes after a visit with Mitch and Cathy, we would continue on to Bish Bash Falls, the highest waterfall in Massachusetts. Situated in an expansive state park, being out in nature was a balm to Des. She loved to breathe in the fresh air and look up at a sun-drenched sky. She actually found a favorite spot, a rock jutting out over the river where we would just spend hours just listening to the babble of the water. At that point she was too sick to make the kinds of long trips we had been accustomed to taking, so we made the most of the opportunities we had for shorter, car excursions. But even shorter trips were difficult because Des had so many digestive issues. We had to make frequent stops along the way. Sometimes we made an event out of it and checked into a motel where Des could be comfortable. If the weather was warm and the motel had a pool or hot tub, all the better. Des would make the absolute best out of every situation.

Another of our favorite excursions was to a lovely inn by the sea in Vermont and to a hotel in New Hampshire that had an up-do-date spa. We could relax, enjoy the amenities and the time without stress. For all our trials, life was good, and I seemed able to relax into that and not be in a perpetual state of worry. We felt blessed.

It was just about this time that Des was contacted by a writer from *Fitness* magazine who had heard about her and wanted to do a major article. Des was thrilled.

"Robert! Just think! What a great opportunity this is for me to make a contribution...to show people that they can deal with cancer in a way that doesn't rob them of the other parts of their lives. This is so terrific!" Her eyes danced with excitement at the prospect.

My mind raced. How could she give a meaningful interview without knowing all the things she had previously not wanted to know?

"Yes, that would certainly be a great forum for you," I said, kind of stalling. Before I could gather my thoughts to say anything more, Des pre-empted me.

"I've thought a lot about it, and in order to really communicate what I need to, I'll have to know what my diagnosis was." She paused. "I'll have to know everything."

Have to know everything... One of Des's greatest coping mechanisms, up until this point, was that she hadn't known all of the details, hadn't wanted to fill her mind with things that she considered irrelevant to her healing, things that would interfere with her ability to cope...things that she had left me to wrestle with.

This was a 360-degree turnaround, but she seemed totally at ease.

I was anything but.

"Are you sure?" I asked, half-hoping she would say she's changed her mind. But she hadn't.

"I'm sure," she answered with a confident smile.

"At this point, she was as insistent about knowing as she had previously been about not knowing.

"I've got to know, Robert," she said, looking at me resolutely. "It's the only way I'll really be able to use the article as a forum to help other cancer patients."

It took me a moment to gather myself. On the one hand, it would be a relief to unload the burden and share some of the specifics. I had carried this for such a long time, and she was, after all, a doctor, and a damned good one, so any ideas about treatment she might have would be valuable. On the other hand, not knowing had been such an important tool for her, and I did not want to damage that in any way.

She sat quietly and listened, looking at me with big sad eyes as I delineated the details of her disease and all she had been through. She learned that the initial tumor was large - 6 centimeters by 4 centimeters - the size of an egg (she had not known the size)... that it was stage 3 breast cancer at that time (she had not known the staging designation)...that 11 of the 12 lymph nodes that were removed were affected (she had not known the number of lymph nodes)...that after two mastectomies and all the punishing chemo she had had, the cancer had still metastasized and created two lesions in her liver (she had only known about one).

To be honest, by that point she had metastases in her bones and a questionable "shadow" in her lung, but that would not have added anything with respect to the story. So I shared only what I thought was relevant and would keep her coping mechanisms intact. I knew she would feel ok with the cancer having never left the liver, and that was what I was going to paint for her.

"I suspected as much," she said, shaking her head. "My God, Robert. What an awful burden I've put on you all these years. I am so, so sorry."

And then she said something that shook me to my core.

"You should have left me."

My body trembled as I watched tears escape from her eyes and roll down her cheeks, desperately trying to keep my own tears in check.

"You really should have left me," she said again.

For me, that had never been an option. "I told you long ago that we are in this together," I said, holding her close. "For today, tomorrow, forever. You are my life and that is all that matters."

We had entered unknown terrain. I buried my face in her hair and just let the tears fall. I had never wanted her to know what she felt she had no need to know. To be honest, I did feel somewhat relieved, but on the other hand, even though it had been enormously difficult for me, I knew I was providing her a type of comfort being the keeper and that allowed her to maintain her faith, and I never wanted her to lose that faith. Ever.

Despite everything she now knew – and perhaps even more so because of it - Des was really looking forward to the *Fitness* interview, and on the following day, armed now, with all the information, Des handled the questions with ease and a kind of purposefulness that I would come to see more and more. She was a woman on a mission, and it was yet another stepping-stone to her formal immersion into palliative care.

The article came out in October 2005 and featured a gorgeous, full page color picture of Des looking happy and healthy. The headline: "I got cancer at age 30..." followed with: "Desiree Pardi was a young, healthy third-year medical student until the unexpected diagnosis that changed her life."

I was terrified that learning the extent of her illness and having all of her colleagues learn the same thing would set her back, but it didn't. On the contrary, it helped to define her goals even more. Yes, it was possible to lead a productive, purposeful life while dealing with serious illness - a message she would go on to communicate with passion for the rest of her career.

She had changed so much, but our families and some of our friends did not quite understand who she was becoming. Looking back, it was understandable, because she had put up such huge guardrails to protect herself from negativity of any kind. There was lots of handwringing by her mother and mine as well, and that just drove Des nuts. It was not the positivity that she both wanted and needed around her and as difficult as it was to make the decision, we began distancing ourselves, more and more, from both families. I was thrilled to see her blossoming into quite an amazing force, and I certainly didn't want to see her knocked off track by well-meaning but unknowingly negative remarks or gestures. Nor did she. Anyone who didn't understand our choice...anyone who brought us down, friends or family, had to be distanced, and the number of people this applied to started adding up. Most of our social activities revolved around her friends who understood and never deviated and that was good, because in the event she really was coming close to the end, I wanted her to be with people with whom she was truly comfortable.

While Des still had the companionship of people at work, and the wonderful, supportive, sister-like friendship she and fellow young doctor Lauren Schwartz had formed, for me this meant more and more isolation. With the exception of my childhood friend Dave, still my best friend after so many years, and his partner Daryl, there were few people who "got it" and with whom I felt comfortable. On the one hand, Des and I were in this together. On the other, I was in this alone, and it was often a terrifying place to be.

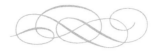

Chapter 25

I had always promised Des that we would celebrate her 40th birthday with a long trip to Europe. While I loved surprising her, I had a feeling her continued love of India probably changed her idea of a European trip, and I was right. When I asked her where she would like to go, she said without hesitation, "Robert, I want to spend my actual birthday at Amma's Peedam. What if we do Rome and then fly over to Amma?"

I, of course, would have said yes to anything, regardless of my fear that she was weakening and it would be dangerous to be so far away from home.

After responding, "Whatever you want Baby," I was rewarded with her signature jumping up and down like a little girl and a great big kiss.

This was going to mark our fifth trip to India, and she pleaded with Dr. Gaynor to do everything he could so that she could be as strong as possible for her 40th. As I look back, I wonder if she knew that it might be her last. Whenever we traveled, Des took care not to disrupt her treatment schedule and we often jumped on the plane the very next day after chemo. She used to joke about how well she slept on board. I, on the other hand, never did, always worried about something going wrong. I marveled at her ability to move forward like that, to have such faith that all would go well, while I could think only about contingency plans in the event that things went south. Yet, this time, her chemo schedule took a backseat and Mitch lovingly accommodated her request.

That evening, on our way to JFK, the smile on Des's face could have rivaled any child's in anticipation of what Santa might bring on Christmas Day. On the plane, she fell into a peaceful sleep, eager to get going the moment we arrived in Rome the next morning. We checked into the Eden, our favorite five-star hotel near the Via Veneto, the boulevard made so famous by "La Dolce Vita." It was October and the weather was just cooling down from summer and settling into those sun-filled but crisp days that make autumn such a spectacular time of year, especially in Rome. We took long walks by the Tiber, lunched *all'aperto* in the Borghese Gardens, drank *apertivi* at the café on the top of The Spanish Steps, and ate great food in cafes along the ancient, narrow streets in the *Trastevere and Testaccio*. It was wonderful to celebrate part of Des's birthday week in Italy and see her so happy, but I couldn't stop myself from thinking, "*How many more birthday celebrations would the future hold?*"

We had a wonderful time and as much as Des loved Rome, it was the second part of the trip that she had really been relishing. It was the prospect of helping people in need that filled Des with such excitement. She said more than once, after planning the trip, how much she desired to give a gift back to the world for the wonderful life she had been given.

After a 14-hour flight, we arrived in Chennai Airport. Des lit up the moment we disembarked, looking perfectly rested after having slept like a baby during the flight. As we moved along and were jostled by the colorful crowds, you would have thought that there was not a thing in the world wrong with her - that she was just a happy tourist about to see things she had only read about in books. Her eyes always gleamed when she saw all the women in their saris. "Robert, I'll never get tired of looking at those wonderful colors! I just love them! It is one of the many things I love about the Peedam honestly — that I have dress traditionally Indian."

"Me too. I can't wait to see you in one of those wrap-around things," I said.

"I'll bet!" she laughed, squeezing my hand. "But I know you just like un-wrapping me."

That was certainly true. Even with all the indignities her body had endured, I still thought she was the most captivating and beautiful woman in the world.

We quickly navigated the chaos of the Chennai airport. It was as if we were whisked through by the divine winds of grace, a stark contrast to our first trip to India, a few years before, when we nearly didn't make it into the country.

God, do I remember that first trip so vividly. How could I forget? The oppressive heat. The waiting for what seemed like hours in the press of an enormous number of people. The heart-stopping moment when we finally arrived at passport control. The official, after thumbing through the pages, looked back at us. It was not a welcoming look.

"Your passports seem in order, but you have no visas, sir," he said sternly.

Des and I looked at each other. No visas! Our perfect planning had not been so perfect after all. I had assumed that as Americans, we would have been able to get our visas at the airport, just like in Dubai. I was always so thorough about everything. How could I have screwed up that way? I was beyond angry at myself.

"I'm a physician," Des calmly said. "My husband and I are expected at Amma's Peedam, near Vellore. We're going to assist with patient care and doctor training at the hospital".

The immigration officer looked at us skeptically. "How do I know this is true?"

Des looked at me for a second then reached in her bag and pulled out a copy of *Fitness* Magazine. The issue with our article had come out the day we left, and we brought it along to show to Dr. Gaynor. She quickly flipped to the piece.

"Here," Des said, waving it at him. "See...this is me, Dr. Pardi."

The man smiled. "Very nice photo miss, but you still need a visa!"

I couldn't believe that some procedural snafu was going to keep us from getting into the country. Des had heard so much about the Peedam and about what Amma was doing for people there and she was so anxious to contribute. I was so irritated with myself. To be honest, the real anger came from my hope, that when we meet Amma, somehow Des would be magically healed. I had to find a way to get her to see him. It was time to pull out the cancer card.

"But we're here to help the Indian people, sir!" I said. "My wife is contributing her time, her expertise. Do you realize my wife has cancer and she travelled all the way to India to donate her time? Can you understand that commitment? We are not here as tourists. She must see Amma," I said rather loudly.

Then, out of the blue, providence intervened. A sharply dressed official, clearly of a higher rank, walked over to us.

"What's all this?" he asked.

"My wife is a doctor, sir, and we are on our way to Amma's hospital in Thirumalaikodi," grateful I was able to get out the impossible-to-pronounce name of the town.

"Amma! A gift from The Divine. Blessed be her name!" he said, using the feminine attribution we had learned that her followers used, believing that Amma was a feminine spirit in a male incarnation. While we had initially had trouble with the concept, it had come to be less of an issue as time went on.

"Give me those passports!" he commanded the other man. "I will take care of the visas here and now."

Des and I both sighed with relief. Disaster was averted. In this part of the world, Amma was a rock star.

So we got our visas and were personally escorted to the car that Amma's people had sent for us. It was kind of an SUV, and it seemed to be in pretty good shape. We couldn't say as much for anything else during the trip, however. The relative calm and modernity of the airport soon gave way to roads under construction, scores of people on rickety bicycles, lopsided, ox-drawn carts, motorcycles, honking horns, crazy drivers, people hanging out the sides of buses, garbage in piles on the sides of the streets, roaming chickens, wild pigs, scrawny dogs, and, of course, wandering, sacred cows. Each time a cow moved into traffic, everything had to stop to let it pass. It amazed us that the cows were never hit, in that they often wandered into incoming traffic.

The roadsides were lined with patched-up shacks and what seemed like hordes of malnourished people. And the smell, was a mix of cooking spices mixed with the stench of refuse. It was hard to breathe. Where were all the profits from the Indian automotive, pharmaceutical, and steel industries — not to mention those call centers where the workers speak English with that particular musical intonation? How could a country function at this level?

I had been very circumspect about the trip to begin with, as what I had read about the country's hygiene and cleanliness left a lot to be desired. What I was seeing, on that first trip, totally justified my apprehensions. But Des had been so adamant and so excited, of course I gave in. But it was awfully hard to conceal what I really thought.

"Robert, isn't this amazing? I can't wait to get to the Peedam. Mitch said I might even be able to give a presentation to the nurses. I can't believe what gifts have come to us since the diagnosis."

That enthusiasm played back in my mind as the squalor of what we were seeing again assaulted me. I remember having held back my immediate agreement, that day, and saying "Baby, I think it's great, but I don't know. India's a third world country and what if something happens? Don't you think we're taking too big of a risk?"

"Remember Auntie Mame?" She quickly responded. "'Live. Live. Live!' And besides, Mitch will be there, and you know he will look over me like his little chickee, just like you do. Don't worry. It will all be OK. The rewards are worth the risks - just like when we moved to Arizona right after we got married."

As unsettled as I was about it, part of me needed her to see this "guru" with the hope —an intense one — that Amma, whose persona we had both come to respect if not actually worship from afar, could really be a divine entity — and lead to a mystical divine cure.

I was far into the stage of praying for miracles. I had already crawled on my knees for her in Fatima, taken her to drink the water of Lourdes, ushered her through all the *porte* for the Jubilee, and had her swim with Dolphins. But maybe this was what I had been searching for.

Despite Des literally having had chemo 24 hours before arriving in India that first time, she was raring to go. She seemed to be super-charged, and nothing could knock her down. She had looked forward to that original trip with its modest accommodations, regimented food, and a practically dawn-to-dusk schedule, all of which couldn't have been more different from the dozens of luxurious trips we had taken during our years together. For days leading up to our departure, she kept saying what an amazing experience it was going to be.

And it was.

At first glance, the Peedam looks like a summer camp but with monkeys and elephants. There are simple white stucco buildings set on nicely manicured areas of green surrounded by mountains in the distance. But looking beyond the immediate area, it is a great deal more than that. It's a very large compound with a magnificent temple, exceptional hospital, gardens, schools, a nursing college, and a food hall that feeds thousands of people a day.

One of the first things we did during our stay was to help feed the people who came to the large food hall for their one meal of the day. Each person sat on the floor in front of a banana leaf, which functioned as their plate. I held the bucket and Des spooned out rice and dhal - a stew made from lentils, peas, or beans. Some of the recipients reached out to touch Des's sunny blonde hair. Others, upon being offered food, offered it back as a sign of gratitude. One woman said to her, "This is not my meal. This is God's food, and as God gives it to me, I should offer it back to others."

Every time we had done this, it put lumps in both of our throats. Here were men, women, and even children, clearly undernourished and lacking in comforts we take for granted, beyond grateful for what they were receiving. It is probably the most sobering experience either of us had ever had. They had such humility, such gratitude in the face of a kind of poverty neither of us had ever encountered. And they didn't seem to rebel against it. They accepted it. Their purpose in life was to connect to The Divine, and they were grateful for everything. The people were extraordinary. Des fell in love with them on our very first visit and fought to keep the tears from falling each time she had the experience.

When we got back to our room, she cried and cried, in awe of the beauty of these people who had such gratitude for what they had and had such a strong belief that, despite the situation they found themselves in, their purpose was to be thankful and to connect to the Divine.

"There's a reason we're here, Robert, a reason all of this happened. I'm meant to learn from my problems and to share what I've learned with others. It's a gift! I've been given an amazing gift. It's so clear that palliative care is the right place for me to be." She reached over to hug me. "And I am so grateful that you have been and continue to be here to help me."

It seemed like ages ago when I had been told her time was running out and needed to convince her to see Dr. Gaynor. Now, here she was, vital and thriving and once again, putting her extraordinary gift of empathy and seemingly boundless energy into helping others. The moment was nearly overwhelming for me.

"Of course I will help you," I managed to get out. "With every breath I take."

We just sat, embracing each other, for a very long time before going back out to join the others, a handful of westerners who had also come to help at Peedam and, of course, the Gaynors who were so happy to share the experience with us. We attended the religious ceremonies which, by this point, were not alien to us. But it was all taken to the next level because it was Amma herself, bathing the idols, greeting the gods, and doing the pujas.

Our first meeting with Amma was truly otherworldly. She was the manifestation of peace and calm. Her wisdom, insights, and teachings were more than impactful. They were truly shifting. There genuinely was something mystical about everything. Personally, I felt great paradigm shifts, and whenever I looked over at Des to assess how she was handling everything, I realized she must had already experienced these shifts. There was no awe on her face, just deep concentration, admiration, and understanding. I was playing catch-up. She had already evolved to a much greater consciousness that I was only just then approaching.

"Service," Amma explained, "is our purpose on earth," And in that philosophy, she certainly had found a devotee in Des. One of the most important things Des did on our trips was to help the doctors there understand levels of patient pain and how to deal with it — an area of medicine in which they were apparently lacking. She came away from that experience with the profound belief that no matter where we are born or what our life circumstances are, we are all the same.

Many of the doctors she interacted with did not speak English very well and yet, using facial expressions and body language, Des was able to communicate her message. It proved to be a pivotal experience for her. The patients she saw were not accustomed to referencing their pain, and it made her think about patients back home. There are so many different cultures among the sick in a big hospital in New York, and she felt she needed to rethink the way they were being handled.

"These people have taught me so much," she said, early on. "Being able to communicate — really communicate — to patients is such a valuable tool. I never realized how differently people from various cultures communicate. Think of all the ethnic groups we have in New York. This is major!" She smiled with true joy on her face. "I'm so grateful to be learning this." Des brought this knowledge back home with her and it helped enrich her practice of pain and palliative care medicine for the rest of her career.

Through the years, we saw the Peedam grow and grow into an extraordinary center for both the spiritual and physical care for thousands upon thousands of India's neediest people. In addition to the hospital and nursing college, Amma built facilities that provided food, clothing, housing, and even textbooks for six government orphanages. She also built a large, six-pointed spiritual center that enlightens with messages not only from the Gita, a Hindu scripture, but from the Bible and the Koran as well. This star serves as a pathway to a huge, glittering golden temple that draws more than 12,000,000 people every year, making it the most visited shrine in the world.

Des glowed working in the hospital, and I found joy working in the food hall. It was an experience that taught me so much about gratitude and service. And like Des had experienced, I too was in awe of these people who were so willing to gift back to me the one meal of the day that they might have. Astonishing.

Now here we were again. After a glorious week in Rome, we returned to Amma's Peedam to celebrate Des's 40th birthday.

Nothing on the roads had changed. It took nearly two hours to drive to the Peedam. Our driver seemed to mistake the horn for the brakes as did most of the other drivers on what passed as a road. We were constantly weaving in and out of traffic in a noisy game of chicken that had our hearts in our mouths the entire way. Even though we had seen it several times before, we still found what we saw out of the window riveting.

It had been a very comfortable flight from Rome compared to the then 20-hour direct flight we were accustomed to from JFK. Regardless, we were relieved to arrive at our destination and plunk down on our bed for a little rest. Des's enthusiasm hadn't waned, but her energy level was not what it had been when we had first arrived at the Peedam many years ago, and it only fueled my fears that we did not have much time left.

Amma, of course, knew that Des was very sick, and every time she said "Amma will take care" I prayed desperately for it to mean spontaneous healing. We had grown to love Amma and feel a peace and serenity in the chanting, participating in her pujas, and being in her presence. On the one hand, it had initially been awkward because of our Catholic upbringing and yet, on the other hand, it all felt right and natural, and we were profoundly grateful to Amma for enriching our lives.

Amma did, in fact, "take care" in many ways over the years and for Des's birthday provided her with the ultimate gift. She performed an extremely special private puja at her house that clearly took Des to another place where she was "on the other side" and experienced total peace.

"It can't get much better than this," Des said, her face glowing with happiness. "Robert, I have never experienced peace like this. Thank you, this is the most amazing birthday I have ever had outside of you proposing to me. I love the life we have created, Robert. I truly do."

My heart nearly burst with gratitude at that moment. I try to keep that memory close. I call on it whenever I forget that through it all, whatever life throws at me, I need to be in a place of gratitude.

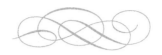

Chapter 26

S oon after, Des was named Chief Fellow in Pain Management
and Palliative Care at Memorial Sloan Kettering, a coveted
position with wide-ranging responsibilities, on both patient care
and academic levels. That Des was selected came as no surprise to
me. She was the most empathetic person I had even met. And her
skills and expertise in pain management and palliative care had
just kept growing and growing. It was remarkable. She kept growing as both a person and a physician. Her colleagues, just about all
of whom, at that point, knew what her personal situation was, were
in awe of her. How in the world had she accomplished all that she
had and keep going with such a loving attitude, such resolve and
sense of purpose? She was extraordinary.

We were doing just about everything that Dr. Gaynor wanted us
to do...the supplements, organic food, green drinks, meditations,
chanting and sound therapy. He monitored Des very closely and
adjusted her chemo treatments with regularity. Even now that she
knew the extent of her disease, she still did not want to know the
specific drugs she was on, and we all respected Des's request, including the chemo nurse who took great care to obscure the drug
names on the bags.

Des was always up and smiling around the other chemo patients. She engaged them in fun conversations about books and
film and shared her knowledge about some of the ways to alleviate
the side effects of the treatments. She was especially happy, one

afternoon, when she was able to help one of her "chemo pals" who was having extreme nausea.

"Ginger," she said enthusiastically. "It will change your life. Promise!"

The next time we met, the woman greeted her with a big smile. "Thank you so much, Desiree. You were right about ginger!"

And she was able to suggest carnitine as an energy booster to another woman and how to ease mouth sores and discomfort with club soda to a third. They loved her for her advice and positiveness - and she loved that she was able to help alleviate pain and discomfort. As sick as she was, she glowed with that knowledge.

I knew enough to know that no matter how well she looked, or how well she seemed to be doing, she was on borrowed time. We never discussed this, nor did I talk to anyone about it. I couldn't bring myself to verbalize it. Somehow, if I didn't dignify it with a name, it would go away.

The following year, 2006, Des was called in for an interview for the post of Medical Director of the new pain and palliative care service at New York Hospital. Everything she had learned and experienced was poised to be put to important and meaningful use. Everything she had been working for was finally in sight.

"Oh my God, Robert. I've just got to get this job," she said, squeezing my hand. "I've got to. I was meant for it!"

I squeezed her hand back, hoping against hope that somehow, someway, she would get the job.

"Remember when Oprah said it was a full circle moment? Well, this is it, Robert. This is where life has been bringing me."

"It is a full-circle moment, isn't it?" I hugged her close.

The position meant so much to her, I wanted her to get it more than anything, but I knew she had a huge hurdle to cross. Chief Resident was one thing, but head of this pivotal new department at one of the most important hospitals in the world was quite another. The decision makers there all knew she was sick, but they also knew how damned smart she was and how committed she was to the practice of palliative medicine. From a qualifications point of view, there was clearly no one on a higher rung. From a health point of view, there was clearly no one closer to bottom.

She went off to the interview that morning filled with confidence, as though there was not an impediment in the world that would keep her from getting the job. "Snoopy," she said as she walked out the door, "everything happens for a reason."

I could barely think until finally the phone rang.

"Well, it went really well, I think. There was a panel of three doctors - I knew them all - and they grilled me pretty thoroughly."

"And?" I interrupted, wanting so much to hear that they had offered her the job on the spot.

"Well, they told me that my background was perfect, of course, but they were searching for someone with more experience. I had to laugh! 'Gentlemen,' I said, 'you might find someone who's had a bit more experience, but I doubt that you'll find anyone who's had more meaningful experience.' Ha! That kinda stopped them cold."

"And?"

"They conferred for a few moments and then one of them said, 'We're going to think about it.' And then I blurted out, 'but I'm ready now!'"

I had to laugh. That was so like Des.

"They said they'd get back to me in a day or so."

The next day for both of us seemed endless. I was anxious, to say the least and Des could always read me. She always made sure to allay my fears, no matter what the scenario. Her optimism was ever present.

"Stop worrying, Robert. I'll get it. I just know I will."

And she did!

The next morning she phoned me from the hospital. "I got it! I got it!" There was so much joy and excitement in her voice. I wished I had been there to share it with her. Frankly, I was flooded with relief. *Thank God it had worked out. Thank God!* "I'm so proud of you, Baby. So proud! We have to celebrate!" I said immediately. "I'll come over and take you to lunch."

"Lunch! Sorry...no time. I have to get back to work in two seconds, but not to worry. I have that Nutella sandwich you made for me. We'll celebrate tonight."

Of course, I was disappointed but agreed. "OK. Tonight. Where would you like to go? The sky's the limit."

"To be honest, I'd really like to stay home. Make me some of your grandmother Mary's rigatoni and I'll be in heaven."

Rigatoni? I would have made her pheasant under glass, if that's what she had asked for. I had been so worried that her illness would work against her, but perhaps the doctors who made the hiring decision didn't know that she was probably in more trouble than they thought - and certainly in more trouble than she, herself, thought. I knew what we were dealing with because every time Dr. Gaynor changed her meds, I knew he was shopping for more time. But for now, she had the time, and she had the job she so desperately wanted, and for that, I was profoundly grateful.

Des's hours at the hospital were long and I did everything I could to ease the burden for her. I had been totally running our household for some time and I was also caring for our new puppy Duncan, who had called out to Des one afternoon as we were passing a pet shop in Midtown Manhattan. Just as I had known we were in trouble years before when Des slowed down in front of that pet store in Arizona and we walked away $1000 poorer and with that big ball of fluff Dollar$ in her arms, I knew this frisky, little Yorkshire Terrier who jumped and scratched and licked the window when he saw Des, would jump right into Des's heart the minute she saw him.

"Oh, Robert. He's soooooo cute!"

Uh, oh. There was no way I was going to say no to anything that would make her happy.

"Let's bring him home Baby."

She flung her arms around me and said over and over "I love you, I love you, I love you Robert Pardi."

"What'll we call him?" I asked.

We were out the door with Duncan in short order. Des wanted to name him Bumbles, because he kind of bumbled along, with a funny gait, but I wanted him to have a manly name like Duncan, after Duncan MacLeod, the immortal from "The Highlander". Des let me win that one - not that she let me win many! And although I always laughed at his funny little walk, I never regretted buying him for Des. He gave her so much joy, rushing to the door when she came home from work, sitting on her lap when she put her feet up to relax, catching the eye and admiration of just about everyone on the street when we took him out for walks. It was the best $1500 I ever spent.

Staff in Des's office was sparse, so I also spent time there helping her with administrative chores...making copies, typing, filing - anything I could do to lighten her load. My dealings with my own office in Dubai, however, had become just about non-existent. My partner was a saint. When we did speak, business rarely came up. It was Des's well-being that he asked about. Our friendship superseded commerce, and for that I was and always will be beyond grateful.

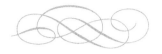

Chapter 27

No matter how busy Des was, she always made time for meditation. It grounded her and gave her peace. The fact that she was able to be peaceful in the face of her illness was a blessing. Her sense of spirituality had grown so much as a consequence of our regular attendance at monthly pujas and most certainly by our life-changing trips to India.

In the past, Des had always liked nice things and no matter what our budget constraints may have been, I had always found a way to get them for her. But as the months went by, she seemed to care less and less about material things. What happened that Christmas was telling.

I was still operating on the "everything and anything I can buy for her to make her happy" track and I saw an exquisite white mink coat and pictured how wonderful it would look on her. Des had to have it, I decided, so I bought it for her as a special surprise for the holiday.

She seemed really excited when, as Christmas Eve turned to Christmas day, she opened the box.

"Oh, Robert. It's beautiful, absolutely beautiful." She lifted the coat from the box and felt the soft fur with her cheek.

I couldn't wait to see it on her. "Let's see how absolutely wonderful it looks!" I said as I helped her put it on. And it did look wonderful on her, complimenting her eyes and her skin. But when I tried to get her to look at herself in the mirror, she was reluctant.

"Oh, let's save that for tomorrow, she said sweetly. "Now let's just snuggle in and celebrate being able to have this Christmas together."

She was right, of course. Being together was what really was important, but she did wear the coat on Christmas day and got lots of ooh's and aah's when we visited our families. (Our moratorium on spending time with our respective families did not extend to holidays.)

We also stopped in to wish "Merry Christmas" to my friend Dave's family. When Dave's mom admired the coat, Des immediately invited her to try it on.

"Really?" Rita Boylan asked?

"Really." Des answered. "Let's see how it looks on you."

Mrs. Boylan put on the coat and dashed to the mirror to see herself. Des followed her. "Do you like it?"

"Oh my God. It's gorgeous," Mrs. Boylan said, running her hands up and down the front of the coat.

"It looks really nice on you," Des said and then looked over to me with a sparkle in her eye. I knew the direction this amazing woman was going. And without fail I was right and watched everyone's jaw drop.

"I want you to have it," she said.

Dave's mom looked shocked. She shook her head. "Oh, no. Desiree...I couldn't..."

"But you can. I want you to have it," Des insisted. "I promise you, it gives me more joy to see how happy it makes you than I could ever have wearing it myself."

The moment she suggested that Mrs. Boylan try on the coat, I had a feeling she was going to do that and my heart nearly burst with joy seeing Des react that way. She had moved to a place in her heart that few of us could ever reach. She had found another way of relating to life. To her, it was now all about joy and sharing. This had become her path, and to see the joy on her face as she made this gift was the best Christmas present I had ever had.

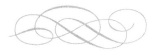

Chapter 28

When I picked up the phone on that late winter morning in March 2008 and heard Mitch Gaynor's voice, my body went numb. Mitch never phoned. When it came to anything social, Des and Cathy did all the planning. When it came to anything medical, Mitch discussed it with me while Des was getting chemo during our regular office visits. Now, in a sedate voice, he said he wanted me to come to his office, alone, to review the results of Des's most recent tests. I could barely get the words out to ask when.

"Whenever you can," he said. "I'll see you as soon as you can get here."

I'm not sure how I got myself to his office. It was only about nine blocks from our apartment and always an easy walk, but I felt as if there was lead in my shoes. The fact that I was in shorts and had forgotten to wear a jacket didn't even register as the cold wind ripped into my torso and stung my eyes. I was already numb. I was blanketed with fear.

When I arrived at the office, there were a couple of people in the waiting area. Dr. Gaynor's assistant and his nurse were both busy on the phone, but as they looked up, I could see sadness in their eyes. I struggled to keep myself together as I nodded "hello" and took a seat, struggling to hold back a barrage of tears.

After a few minutes, Mitch, as we both had come to call him, came out and asked me to join him in his office. He ushered me in and quietly closed the door. I could barely walk the few feet to sit in the chair opposite his desk, tears ready to break through my will to stay strong. He leaned forward to speak, but before he could say anything, words tumbled out of my mouth. "I know what you're going to tell me," I said. This was a conversation I had known for a long time we would one day have...a conversation that I never allowed myself to rehearse, because maybe if I didn't let the words form in my head, they would never have to come out of my mouth...a conversation that maybe at that point, I could magically make evaporate if I somehow got the words out first.

Mitch lowered his head for a long moment then looked back up and said, "The cancer has become uncontrollable."

There it was: *uncontrollable.* For years we had matched wits with the disease, parrying back with its every thrust. A couple of years before, Mitch had literally saved Des from impending death when, unbeknownst to everyone, a chemotherapy drug that she had previously been on was putting her in cardiac arrest. The recognition that this was happening came to him while he was doing a puja. The very next morning, he had a noted cardiologist confirm it with tests. Mitch had saved her then and had kept on saving her. He had given her the past three years...three really good years filled with joy, purpose, and thankfulness, and the time to accomplish so much.

Uncontrollable. Des had dazzled colleagues with her knowledge and zeal and her unique ability to steer patients through their most difficult days. She had inspired hundreds of students to look ahead to their days as physicians with an expanded consciousness. She had won numerous awards and her publishing credits fill page upon page. On top of her professional accomplishments, she had run pink ribbon races to raise funds for cancer - the one activity she had been involved in with her mother, sister, aunt and some friends that was clearly "breast cancer" and a departure from her posture of not wanting to dwell on it, and especially not wanting her mother to dwell on it. She also sang in a church choir and played Auntie Mame to our niece Jess, my brother Michael's then seven-year-old daughter, taking her shopping and sight-seeing and showing her how to luxuriate for an afternoon with a delicious manicure and pedicure at an upscale spa. She also loved to spend time with her sister's daughter, but it was much less frequent.

We had enjoyed dinners and laughter with those friends we had kept close - David and Daryl, Lauren, and Phyllis, who, amid gales of laughter, we got to know in the treatment room in Mitch's office. And there were the nights at Lincoln Center watching opera from her favorite first-ring, center seat...and the nights at home, that we both relished, polishing off some baked ziti, then snuggling up to "30 Rock," "How I Met Your Mother," and "Saturday Night Live" on TV, like any normal couple.

There were also our trips to India, weekends at Bish Bash Falls and frequent getaways to Florida, so that Des could have a couple of days of the sun and sea she loved so much. And there had been her 40th birthday celebration.

Uncontrollable. Please, God, don't let that birthday be her last. I'll do anything, God. Anything.

"What can I do, Mitch?" I asked. "Anything, Mitch, anything. What can I do...?"

How hard it must have been for him to answer me, this loving doctor who had become a close medical colleague to Des and such a dear and close friend to us both.

Mitch looked away for a second then back at me, and in a soft, measured voice said, "Normally, we would put her in hospice care."

Hospice? Dear God, that means she has a maximum of six months...

"But," he went on, "that would never be right for her."

"Never," I agreed, shaking my head. "Never, she wants to go until she can't, until her body just gives out. What can we do? What can I do? Mitch, please anything, I will do anything."

"You'll have to be her hospice," he said. "You'll have to give up everything and just take care of her."

At that point, I'd already pretty much done that, happily, willingly, with all my heart, but I know what he was asking me was to cross the line. The line between husband and caregiver would become blurred. I would need to perform medical tasks.

"Of course," I said. "I will do anything, just show me, teach me what to do. But you know Des, we have to ensure she can do her job for as long as she can."

"And that's what she should do, for as long as she can. We both know what her work means to her."

There was a long silence.

"I don't think we should mention any of this to her," I said. "Do you?"

Mitch shook his head, then my friend, this gifted doctor to whom we owed so much, embraced me. I tried to be strong - I really did - but I could not stop the tears. This was the day I never wanted to come...the day I somehow thought I could stave off in-definitely...the day when I would have to muster up every ounce of strength I had to go forward cheerfully and purposefully and help Desiree live every last moment that she would have on this earth in the way that only she knew how.

"You can do this," Mitch said, patting me on the back. I could see that he was struggling to keep his composure.

I walked out of his office into the reception area. His nurse and assistant were both in tears as they came to embrace me. No words were spoken. They were not necessary. They had both been of enor-mous support, comfort and help the last three years. I kissed them both, stood for a moment, then turned to leave. I slowly opened the door and a gush of frigid air hit me as I plunged into the late winter afternoon.

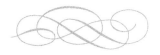

Chapter 29

Our lives continued much as they had the previous several months. I had long since given up anything but the most fundamental contact with my company in Dubai. Des had become the absolute center of everything. I had become fanatic about managing everything that concerned her well-being. I also started taking her to work in the morning in a taxi in addition to picking her up at night, accompanied by Duncan, who always made her smile. But my over-protectiveness sometimes grated on her.

"Robert, you're smothering me," she said, clearly annoyed. "I'm a big girl, you know."

"I know you are, but I enjoy taking you to work and picking you up. Are you going to deprive me of that?" I joked.

She shook her head and rolled her eyes. "Yeah," she said. "Like I have any choice."

I know she was finding my caretaking oppressive, but she tolerated me. She knew it was helping her carry out her purpose, her passion, to care for others. She knew I would stop at nothing to help her be as productive as possible for as long as she could, even at the risk of getting on her nerves.

As if to punctuate the irony of it all, just a few weeks after Mitch and I had the conversation, Des received the New York Hospital's Patient Centered Care Award, an honor given to a physician, across disciplines, who was recognized for putting patients first. I was proud of her, of course, but so wished that, at this point, she would put herself first. Maybe if she did, it could buy us a few more months...

She seemed to be doing well, and even though I knew Mitch was correct in his prognosis - he would never have even uttered the word "hospice" if he weren't 100 per cent sure. I hoped against hope he was wrong.

Spring came and went and miraculously, Des seemed to be stable. Then, one day in the height of the summer heat, she suggested that we take our niece Jess to Boston for a weekend. It was one of Des's favorite cities and Jess had never been there. Des thought it would be fun to walk The Freedom Trail, have proper afternoon tea near Copley Square, and ride the swan boats in The Public Garden. Since she seemed to be holding her own, I didn't want to veto the idea.

We picked Jess up in Long Island and drove the six hours to Boston. This was the first time Jess had ever been on an overnight away from her parents, and she was so excited. Des was excited, too. She loved being with our niece and seeing how the three of us being together made Jess so happy. As for me, as much as I loved them both, for weeks I had been fighting with myself, trying not to tick off those months and weeks in my head, counting the precious days we might have left together. Des had long ago embraced living in the moment. I was not quite there, but I was determined to get there so I could share that sensibility with Des. I made up my mind to succeed on that trip, because I knew my time frame was not open-ended.

We arrived at our hotel and Jess was thrilled. We had booked adjoining rooms, so she would be near us. She had never been in a hotel room before and she explored every nook and cranny.

"I feel just like Eloise!" she said with a huge giggle.

"But you're prettier," Des said, hugging her close.

I grabbed my camera and snapped a photo of my two favorite girls looking so happy being together. It's a wonderful photo - a very special moment in a wonderful day.

We toured the city, had a nice dinner in one of Boston's famous seafood restaurants, and turned in early. We had packed in a lot in a long day, and both Des and Jess were tired.

"Aunt Des," Jess said, "Can we keep the door between the rooms open?"

Des laughed. "Of course we can, honey. Uncle Rob and I are just a hug away." And there were lots of hugs, that night. Lots.

The next morning, we boarded a tour boat for a whale watching expedition. We left from the harbor and spent hours in the ocean waters close to the city. We watched the humpbacks jump and dive, their fan-like tails dancing over the waves. These amazing creatures, which we sadly learned are unfortunately becoming endangered, are generally about 50 feet long and weigh an amazing 37 tons. Jess was wide-eyed, and Des was clearly so happy to be able to provide the experience for her. I looked at them...Des standing behind Jess, with the sun illuminating the joy on her face, and I drank in the moment. It was a day filled with such moments, each and every one precious, and finally I was doing it - living in the moment.

But the joy didn't last. About 1 AM, that night, Des woke me. "Robert, you need to get me to a hospital," she said quietly. "I feel like I am dying."

Through all she had endured the last several years - the pain, the procedures, the endless chemotherapy - I had never heard Des say anything like that...and armed with the information I had about her prognosis, my heart just about stopped. *Please, God, don't let it be now. Please...*

I leaned over and felt her forehead. She was burning up.

"It's probably another neutropenic fever," she said. "But this one's really bad. Better get me to the hospital."

Des had had neutropenic fevers before, but she had never couched it in such terms – and I knew these fevers could be fatal. We were very close to a major hospital - just one long block away. I don't know if I had subconsciously picked the hotel because of that, but was glad that I had. Des was too weak to walk, and I was worried that I couldn't carry her that short distance, so I phoned for an ambulance.

We threw on some clothes and I woke Jess.

How in Hell was I going to tell my niece what was going on without scaring her?

"Aunt Des isn't feeling well, honey," I said. "We need to take her to the hospital really fast."

"The hospital?" Jess asked, her eyes filled with fear. "Why?"

"That's the best thing to do when you're on vacation and don't know any doctors," I said. Truth was that Des probably did know some doctors on staff, just as she knew top doctors in many hospitals. She had applied to and been accepted to Brigham and Women's not that many years ago, and some of her classmates had done internships and residencies there.

Jess tiptoed over and peeked through the open door. Des waved faintly to her.

"Get some clothes on now, sweetie," I said. "We need to leave right away."

Jessica and I each held one of Des's hands during the short ride to the hospital. And when we checked Des in, Jess tugged at the sleeve of the on-duty doctor. "Please take good care of my Aunt Des," she said. "You have to make her get better. I love her so much!"

That nearly did me in, but I had to stay strong. I was able to get one of the candy stripers to look after Jess while the doctors in the ER went to work. Des had a 104-degree fever. I didn't know that it was possible to be alive with a temperature that high, let alone at the 106 it hit a few hours later. The staff couldn't believe that someone that sick had been able to travel. They also couldn't believe that Des, with all her training and expertise, didn't want to know specifics and was deferring to me to deal with it all.

The slew of tests they did confirmed what I knew: Des was on the precipice of life. They told me that it was highly doubtful that she would leave the hospital. *You don't know my wife,* I thought.

They flooded Des with mega-dose antibiotics and in the saddest of ironies, offered her Palliative Care. Des, of course, refused. She would handle it her way. She was determined to leave the hospital and get back to work. And I was determined to help her do both. Des insisted I give her the neupogen, a drug that's used to combat the drop in white blood cells that often happens to cancer patients. By then I had become accustomed to carrying it with us whenever we traveled.

"Robert, give me that fucking shot and some Tylenol and get me the hell out of here. If you don't, I will get up and do it myself! They don't know me here. They don't know how I bounce back. They will only see my disease. Give me that fucking shot!"

I agreed with her, but I was scared. I knew the truth, and I was questioning everything.

"Baby, let's just call Mitch first, ok?"

She just huffed and we called Dr. Gaynor and he said to give her neupogen and then called the hospital. He must have explained everything and how she coped because there was no further talk about palliative care visiting. The doctors arrived with a neupogen shot in hand, not knowing we had one with us, and started her on IV Vancomycin. Her temperature dropped almost immediately. I called my brother to come get Jessica, and by the time he and my mother arrived the next day, Des was feeling much better.

"I'm sorry our vacation was cut short, honey," Des said to Jess. "But tell you what - I'll be better soon and we'll do something that's even more fun...like go to Florida and swim with the dolphins. Would you like that?"

"Oh, Aunt Des...that would be so much fun!"

"Uncle Rob took me to do that a couple of years ago, and it was great. I think you'll like it!"

"Oh, I know I will!" Jess said. "So you have to get better fast."

Des waved her a kiss goodbye and I walked my mother, brother and niece down the hall.

"Aunt Des swallowed a bug while we were whale watching," Jess told her father and grandmother. "That's why she's sick."

I hugged her close. If only that had been the case.

But it did appear that for now, we had a reprieve - if just for a short time. The reality of Des's condition was inescapable. It was just not this time.

After four days, Des was chomping at the bit to leave the hospital. She swallowed a huge dose of aspirin to bring down her fever and, against the recommendations of the doctors who were looking after her, discharged herself.

"I've just got to get back to work!" she insisted.

We drove home and, in a few days, Des was, indeed, back at work, teaching, lecturing, and seeing very sick patients.

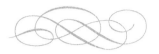

Chapter 30

By the fall of 2008, Des had lost a great deal of weight, dropping from her healthy-looking 125 pounds to an alarming 85. She was extremely fragile. The need to stick to organic and totally healthful foods took a back seat to getting some weight on her. Green drinks and plates full of vegetables gave way to Big Macs, Ben & Jerry's Cherry Garcia, bowls of Count Chocula cereal, Starbucks Frappacinos, Entemann's frosted marshmallow cakes, and of course our traditional caramel apple. I served her anything I could find loaded with calories on a sliver plate. As only Des could do, she took to her new regimen of *verboten* foods with relish.

"Why have you been keeping this stuff from me?" she asked mischievously as she devoured a bacon, lettuce and tomato sandwich loaded with mayo. Then she laughed. "Ok. Don't answer that!"

But even all of that was not enough to deliver the nourishment her body needed to keep going. Every night while she slept, she was fed intravenously with TPN, total parenteral nutrition. I could never sleep, of course. I was fixated on the intravenous liquid making its way into Des's vein, watching the mixture of glucose, amino acids, lipids, vitamins and minerals drip into her body, hoping against hope that every drip would bring her yet another day.

Des ate most of what I put in front of her, and also the almond butter sandwiches I packed for her to eat mid-day at the hospital and to snack on whenever she had a moment. We quickly got her weight back to 115 lbs. and she gained some strength.

But there were days when it was not that easy to get her to eat and she got really angry with me. "I hate you!" she yelled at me one morning. "I wanted a husband, not a parent!"

I steeled myself and tried not to let that penetrate. I knew that I had been a pain in the ass, but I also knew that she was perilously close to a time I didn't want to acknowledge and anything I could do - anything at all, even though it made her angry with me - I would continue to do.

"You have to give me freedom, Robert! You just have to."

I just shook my head. "And you'll just have to put up with me," I said. "I don't enjoy being this way. All I want to do is to ensure you're with me my entire life."

"I know how hard all of this is for you, and I love you more than I even have the words to express it," Des responded, "but I need to feel free in order to feel fully alive...to feel normal. Please help me with this Robert...please. You are more than my caregiver. You are my husband, my lover, my best friend."

We were in a standoff and I didn't want to back down. I heard what she was saying, and I knew in my heart how she was feeling, but my fear was suffocating me. Then she looked at me with those big blue eyes and said, "Robert, I need to live."

That was it, those were the heartstrings to pull. And with that, I started letting go of the reigns and giving her the freedom she was demanding. I had to. It was her life. She had directed her care from the beginning, and I had to give her the choice to direct this stage, regardless of her knowing what was happening or not. I had to do my best to quell my fears and let her live. To let us live the best we could for whatever time we had left. Yes, Dr. Gaynor told me that I had to be her hospice. Yes, he told me I couldn't let down my guard for one moment, lest the worse would happen, but it did not mean that I become her warden. I could give her back her freedom and stay vigilant from the sidelines - and I was going to find a way to do it.

I hoped against hope that she didn't realize her time on this earth was dwindling rapidly, but how could she not? She was one of the smartest, best damned doctors that the medical profession had produced.

As much as I was giving damn near 120 percent of myself, Des needed more and I was lucky enough to be surrounded by a great group of people. One of the most wonderful things about being a patient of Mitch Gaynor and attending his pujas and meditation sessions was getting to know some really remarkable people - people from many countries, ethnicities and professional backgrounds who were regular attendees. Most of them had two things in common: serious illness, usually cancer, and the extraordinary care they received from Mitch. And it was his exemplary care that fostered each of us wanting to help the other. One day, I was talking to a gentleman at puja, who worked in sound therapy, about Des's increasing insomnia.

"John, do you have any ideas of what could help?"

"Let me think about it," he replied with the most caring tone.

A few days later a sound therapy chair arrived at our door with a note saying, "Happy Early Christmas, Santa". The chair was incredible. It vibrated to the music, and massaged her body while she listened to surround sound delta waves to help her sleep and it worked.

A few weeks later Christmas was upon us and Des was in much better condition. We were so thankful for another Christmas together. Even though tensions were high, we planned on seeing our families and buying them gifts, but what Des's greatest concern was getting gifts for some of the nurses she worked with...little things to show them how much she appreciated their help and support.

"The nurses are so great, Robert...so important to patient care, and so, so helpful to me," she said. "I just want to say a little 'thank you.'"

She picked out small items she knew each would appreciate and she wrapped them with Santa Claus paper and bright red bows.

Des beamed as she handed the women and men her small tokens of thanks and respect - and they beamed right back with big smiles and even bigger hugs. It was crystal clear how she felt about them - and how they felt about her.

Des loved Christmas but I was plagued with the reality that this might be her last one. I was determined, however, to banish that thought and help her enjoy every moment of the holiday. We spent Christmas Eve at my Aunt Roe's, and it was wonderful. She had her traditional open house and people came in and out all afternoon and evening. My mother's side of the family was large and Des loved all the people, laughter and good cheer.

"This is how Christmas should be, Robert!" she said, as she snuggled up against me and whispered in my ear.

"Yes," I whispered back. *Yes...*

The next day, Christmas 2008, it was time for Des's family. We had taken on the tradition of hosting Christmas Day because Des was thrilled that we finally had an apartment large enough to do it and she always said that no one made a turkey as good as I did. The turkey and all the trimmings turned out great and it was a mostly good day, marred only with a bit of tension here and there. Des had withdrawn significantly from her family and her sister was hurt. Feelings were bared and an argument broke out between her and her sister. Many people, including my and Des's family, just didn't really understand how and why Des had changed. They didn't comprehend why she needed to retreat from anyone who did not understand how she needed to cope and how it had become paramount to her ability to survive. I still think how hard it must have been for her parents to not be able to talk with her about what was going on. Then again, Des did not know the half of it, or maybe she did by that point.

I stopped the fight and told the family they had to leave. From the look on Des's face, I knew that it was the right course of action.

"Do you know how sick your sister is?" I asked once we were out in the hallway. "Can you understand how much she is going through?" I was seething. "How can you behave this way? Do you realize this could be her last Christmas, *her last Christmas*?"

Des's parents did not say anything. I'm sure they were too upset to speak, and I think they respected my need to vent at that point. Desiree's sister loved her - it was obvious - and she explained to me that she had felt like she was losing Desiree. That she had already lost her sister. That she wanted to help but Des wouldn't let her. I explained that the best way to help her was to let her be, and not try and fix anything.

"None of us had any idea how much time Desiree had left," I said. "None of us, not even me, can truly understand what she thinks and feels, and whatever her coping skills are, we must respect them. This is her journey, and we can't let our emotions interrupt it. We must give her that gift, regardless of the pain and suffering it causes us."

Everyone finally calmed down and Des invited them back into the apartment, but after they finally left and I was cleaning up, Des just sat in the corner, staring out the window.

"What's wrong, Baby?" I asked as I put my arms around her. "Do you want to tell me what happened?"

"No Robert, what happened is not important," she sighed.

She remained silent for a few minutes before continuing. "You know, Robert, I had them come back in the house for my parents," she said, her eyes now welling up. "I don't know how long I will be around and I wanted to spend this Christmas with them. I love them but I can't confront all of this drama anymore." She looked at me resolutely. "When I die, I only want my parents in the room with me. You must ensure that is the case."

I really didn't know what to say. It was the first time I had heard Desiree talk about her death so matter-of-factly, but I had to remove my own worries from impacting my answer. I had to assure her that I would carry out her wishes.

"Of course, Baby. If that moment comes," I said as I kissed her forehead.

Not long after Christmas, Des re-iterated her decision about who she wanted with her when it was her time - just two people... her mother and me and no one else. I didn't much want to discuss it again, primarily because we had made a pact never to talk about death, but she was adamant.

"I even told Lauren," referring to her best friend, "about my decision so that she could support you and so you wouldn't have to be alone policing everything."

At first I was upset that she found it necessary to bring her friend into it. Wasn't I enough? When did I not move heaven and earth to protect her? And then I started worrying. What did she know that I didn't? Was she in pain? But I knew she would change the subject and move on to sunnier topics, so I was left with the gnawing fear that was growing bit by bit by the day.

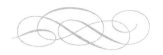

Chapter 31

T hen, as the year turned, our optimism grew. Des received an invitation to speak at a major Visiting Nurse Service meeting to talk about palliative care. She was so excited, and I was thrilled for her.

"Robert," she said, "this is such a big deal! I have so much value to add through this speech." She was absolutely joyous thinking about it. Her whole face lit up at the prospect.

The VNS of New York, which makes more than 2,000,000 patient visits a year, is the oldest and largest not-for-profit health care provider in the US. The standard-bearer for care giving, they are highly regarded by physicians and patients alike, and have a tradition of inviting top-flight physicians to speak at their "grand rounds" events. That Des was excited about giving the speech did not surprise me. What did, however, was how she decided to handle the topic.

"I've actually never thought of myself as a patient," she said, shaking her head with an almost childlike sense of discovery.

I knew, of course, that she really hadn't and my heart clutched. Des had always compartmentalized her experience as a cancer patient...relegated it to a corner, somewhere. It had been one of her greatest coping mechanisms, and because of that she had had the strength and will to forge ahead and accomplish so much.

"When I started to put my thoughts down on paper," she said, "I realized that so much of what enables me to do a good job as a palliative care practitioner is because I have had the experience of being on the other end."

She looked up at me with her beautiful blue eyes, still bright and shining through all that she had endured. "I've not really wanted to think about that...but I guess you know that."

"Guess so..." I said in a near whisper. I really thought I would cry at that moment, but I couldn't do that. I couldn't stop to feel anything that might impede me from helping her make this speech everything it could be, having no idea at that point, how her remarks would be received, how they would come to be known as a "blueprint for palliative care," and how they would also be her legacy.

"It's time to let it in," she said, "to acknowledge that my experience has informed my work as a physician. I've learned so, so much, Robert. It's finally time for me to share what I've learned."

She had come to a pivotal moment, and her face radiated a peaceful resolve. *Surely she knows*, I thought to myself. *Surely...*

I took a deep breath. "Yes," I said softly. "What can I do to help you?"

"Just be there for me, as you have for the last 23 years."

I took her hand and squeezed. "You know that I am here and always will be."

"I know," she said, as she squeezed back. "I really know..."

The morning of the speech, Des seemed happy and confident and exuded a kind of determination that was almost otherworldly. Her eyes sparkled and she seemed unstoppable. It was unusual for her not to have practiced it in front of me, but she hadn't suggested that, and I didn't bring it up. It was unspoken between us but understood: she had to go this one alone.

The room at the VNS headquarters was set up for "grand rounds" speakers. In teaching hospitals, grand rounds traditionally are an opportunity for doctors, residents and medical students to review specifics of a particular case with the patient present and able to answer questions. Over time that has changed and now they are often conducted without the actual patient there. In many instances, such as Des's lecture at the VNS, they have morphed into having an expert in a particular field of medicine address an audience of colleagues and other medical personnel. But this case was different. On this day, the doctor was not only the speaker, she was also the patient.

The VNS Grand Rounds Lecture was particularly well thought of, with experts such as Memorial Sloan Kettering psychiatrist Jimmie Holland and New York Presbyterian's renowned internist and educator Eric Cassell as guests not that long before. These were esteemed colleagues whom Des highly regarded. Her having been invited was, as she enthusiastically put it, a "big deal!"

Although she hadn't fully regained all the weight she had lost, Des looked good that day and I was full of pride as I watched her at the podium from my front row seat. She still had a smile that could light up any room. I looked around at the 75 or so professionals waiting to hear what this very young head of palliative care at New York Presbyterian/Weill Cornell had to say, wondering how many of them knew the extent of her illness.

In moments, they all would.

Did Des know that this was her opportunity to make a real impact on how the medical community viewed palliative care? Of course. But did she also know that this opportunity might be her last one? I think so. During those early weeks of 2009, I think she was in the process of coming to terms with her mortality, and this was her opportunity to leave important and lasting wisdom.

And she did.

"Many of you know, I am sure, that I, myself am a cancer patient," she began. "As my husband Robert, who is here with us today knows, I have never really thought of myself as a patient. Cancer was something I dealt with when I had to and frankly that 'having to' was on quite a regular basis. Nonetheless, I chose to put it in a box...compartmentalize it, as the psychiatrists call it. But it worked well for me, and enabled me to get on with my life, get my PhD and my MD and to become a palliative care physician."

"What I'd like to share with you today is what I call **Walking the Line: Lessons learned from being both cancer patient and palliative care physician.**"

There was a buzz in the audience, but the attendees quickly settled down, and in no time, Des had their total and complete attention.

She began by giving a brief history of her education and the course of her illness. Then she continued with remarks which some in the medical field have said should be required reading for medical personnel, as well as taught in medical schools.

Using a power point, Des explained that, as a patient, she learned the importance of thoughtful communication. "This", she said, "is **Lesson #1 - Bad news does not have to be broken badly.**" She cited that day in Dubai when it was incumbent upon me to tell her that the breast lump the doctors had taken out was indeed malignant. Somehow, I had instinctively conveyed the information to her in a way that didn't instill fear.

"The better the news is broken," Des said, "the better that patient is able to manage their disease. Too often I have seen this not be the case."

"But it is equally as important," she explained that **"The patient not be given false hope, which she likened to poison. This was Lesson #2,"** which she learned because the surgeon who removed the lump in her breast had given her every indication that the lump would be benign. Then, when the results came back malignant, she felt blind-sided.

"This should be avoided at all costs. False hope," she said, "can cause significant harm to both patients and their families. The first thing we in health care have to remember," she reminded everyone, "is first do no harm."

While often offered by well-meaning physicians, she continued, false hope frequently leads patients to make bad decisions, such as opting for painful or debilitating treatments when they might be far better off in choosing hospice care. "This is one of the main reasons I chose the field of palliative care," she said.

I could hear the audience stir on that remark, and I wondered how many sitting there that day had unwittingly been the provider of false hope to patients who were in their care.

At that point she talked about something that I'm sure is very difficult for physicians to determine: **What does the patient want to know?** This was **Lesson #3.** She illustrated that point with her own story and detailed how she had awakened after her lumpectomy in Dubai knowing that not only was it cancerous, but there was lymph node involvement because a PC - an intravenous drug delivery system - was attached to her wrist. "At that moment," she said, "I was sure I was about to die."

Then she looked at me and smiled. "It was my husband Robert who came to tell me the next day that the margins were not clear and that I needed a modified radical mastectomy...not the doctor, but my husband."

That drew quite a stir. I smiled back as I remembered that day more than 10 years before when I, too, thought that our young lives were over, never dreaming that during the next decade Des would be able to meet such enormous challenges - and that together, we would reap such enormous rewards.

But even those in the audience who had previously known that Des was a cancer patient most likely did not know how she went on to handle her disease, choosing not to know many specifics and choosing to put me in charge of much of her care. She explained that when that doctor in Dubai gave the information to me and then I relayed it to her, we both realized that it worked very well for her to have that information that way, filtered through me.

"It allowed my coping mechanisms to remain in place," she said, "the largest of which was denial."

There was a big audience buzz on that remark. It seemed like such a huge admission - and such a brave one. If Des had run it by me, I would have challenged her use of the word "denial," because that in no way told the story. Early on in her illness, she had said to me, "Robert, I need you to handle this because I do not want my knowledge as a medical student and then as a doctor to undermine me. I do not want fear or self-judgment to get in the way of my progress." Des was exercising her right to choose the coping mechanism that worked for her - something that palliative care heartily endorses.

Des went on to detail how this way of doing things was challenged by some medical professionals, but also about how she held her ground until we found a team of doctors that would respect her philosophy and carry out her requests.

"Throughout my schooling and residency training," she said, "I have seen the consequences of patients being forced into hearing information that they did not want to hear. This overwhelmed their ability to cope, leading to severe emotional and existential distress." This had happened to her, she went on to explain, when an oncologist whom I had requested not to detail the specifics of her disease had done just that.

"No one has the right to take away another's coping mechanism without permission," she said. "Patients have a right to be allowed to make that choice. Patients should have autonomy - the right to know, and the right not to know - even when that might be detrimental."

"Asking patients what they want to know is one of the most commonly missed steps in doctor-patient communication. I chose palliative care," she continued, "to help protect other patients who feel just as I do."

This clearly struck a nerve as the audience buzz picked up again. Perhaps they hadn't thought about what a patient might want or not want to know. Or perhaps they were surprised that someone like Des, with all her medical and scientific education and experience, had chosen that path.

I made eye contact with Des at that moment and I could see how excited she was as she realized how well she had driven that point home. It was so important to her. It had been key to her survival, and she needed to share that with colleagues who were in a position to see to it that other patients could also have that autonomy.

She went on to talk about **Lesson #4 - What she had learned from her own physical and emotional symptoms.** She detailed the extraordinary path of treatment she had endured for so many years. I looked_around and saw expressions of surprise, incredulity...pain and empathy. This was a cancer story like none other they had ever heard. She talked about how, after having to wait for nearly a year to re-enter medical school to finish her last two years, many people questioned why she would want to go back. Some, including several people who were close to her, even doubted that she would.

There had never been a question in her mind about continuing her medical education. "I knew more than ever that I wanted to be a doctor. Who better?" she asked, her face lighting up with a big smile.

She also talked about how she was almost relieved when her cancer had recurred and how it had been like the Sword of Damocles hanging over her head. At least, then, she knew. But it also put her into a depression, and she was very up front about that, and how she agreed to go to therapy, against her will, thinking it would be an enormous waste of time.

"I went kicking and screaming," she said, "but, as it turned out, that therapy, more than anything up to that point, saved my life."

There was something in her voice that I recognized - something that no one else in the audience would have picked up...but it was at that very moment when I knew, for certain, that Des knew she was dying. I just knew, and I felt numb, as though all of the blood had been drained from my body, but I had to keep it together. It was more important than ever that I be strong. Our eyes locked and I knew that she felt my love, as I certainly felt hers in return. It's a moment that's carved in my memory, for all time.

She continued with her speech, explaining that, armed with what she had experienced as a patient, she used her new-found sensibility in her work with patients and their families, going to battle again, with her own cancer, including the bout with pain after her liver operation that had her crying out in anguish.

"When a patient tells you they are in pain - listen! When they say it's really bad - listen! I am here to tell you that unbearable pain IS unbearable!"

She paused after that, and let it sink in - and judging by the faces in the group, she had clearly made her point. I doubt that any healthcare worker in that room would ever again give a patient's declaration of pain anything but the most serious attention.

The she moved on to how cancer made her think about death and how switching her care to a gifted, integrative oncologist whose own spirituality led her on a new path had enriched her life in innumerable ways. The audience was absolutely riveted when she talked about her experiences in India.

She even went on to discuss such personal things as her sadness in losing her hair, her embarrassment in dealing with uneven breast sizes, the changes in body image and even issues surrounding sexuality - which made me somewhat uncomfortable, but proud of her that she could share on such an important level.

Her courage dazzled me. When I looked around at the audience, I could see she had dazzled them as well. Their faces registered incredulity, awe and profound respect. And there were several who fought to keep their emotions in check.

And then Des went on to **Lesson #5 - The dangers of empathizing too much.** She reminded the group that it's the patient's moment - not theirs - and that everyone deals with difficult medical experiences in their own way. She rarely broke those rules, she said, but one patient moved her to do so.

One day, she shared, she was called to do a palliative care consultation with a young woman in her early thirties who had had a diagnosis of early esophageal cancer. Her prognosis was excellent, but she would definitely have to undergo chemotherapy, and that left the woman feeling very sorry for herself.

"I won't do chemotherapy," the young woman said. "I'll lose my hair. I'll look awful...I'll have no life," at which point, Des whipped off the wig she was wearing, looked at the amazed patient straight on and said, "Do I look like someone who has no life?"

The woman was dumbfounded, of course, but listened to every word Des had to say and I know she will always be grateful that Des convinced her to go forward with chemotherapy. That woman, today, is in total remission, leading a full, cancer-free life.

Des went on to **Lesson #6 - That it is impossible to do without support.** She told the group how grateful she was to so many who had helped her along the way...professors, classmates and medical colleagues who had been instrumental is allowing her to create school and work schedules that would accommodate her treatments. She was fortunate, she said. Fortunate! "I would not be able to do it without having such wonderful and supportive colleagues, and so **my last lesson is - Be Thankful.**" She singled out many doctors and nurses by name, but closed on how very thankful she was to have Duncan, our Yorkshire Terrier...and to have me.

At that moment, I wanted to leap out of my seat and scream for all the world to hear how thankful I was to have her...to have this amazing woman as my wife, my lover, my teacher, my partner in life, knowing only too well that our journey together was coming to an end. But I just beamed, fighting back tears as I had so many times before when Des did extraordinary things. And I continued to beam at the post-speech brunch when Des was besieged by attendees who expressed their gratitude at having been able to hear her "Lessons". I was this amazing woman's husband. What a gift I had been given.

She barely had a moment to have anything to eat. Just about everyone wanted to chance to talk to Des and to thank her for helping them see things about the practice of medicine that they had never seen before ... to make them realize that palliative care needs to be woven tightly in the everyday practice of medicine ... that patients had to be respected as people, and to be allowed to keep their dignity. Her lessons were life changing, many of them said, and they were so grateful to her.

Des's response to each of them: "I am the one who is grateful to have had the opportunity to share all of this with you!"

It was a singularly wonderful day and I was able to see the enormous impact on the people who were in that room. The doctor who was head of the VNS at the time said that people told him it was the most impactful grand rounds they had ever attended. They were affected not only on a professional level, but on a personal one as well.

"Because she had faced her life and fears so courageously," he later said, "it made them look to life."

Des would have loved hearing that, because no one looked to life more than she had.

The Last Chapter

I always knew I couldn't save Des, but somehow, I thought I could just keep her going. She had survived so much, for so long, that it became our normal. She fell, I helped her get back up and we moved forward again and again ... more slowly and for shorter distances each time, but always forward and always together. Why couldn't it just continue on this way? But of course, it couldn't and just a few months after she gave that landmark speech to that rapt group of medical professionals, Des's all-too-brief but extraordinary time on this earth came to an end. After a short stay at Mount Sinai hospital, where she was placed under the care of Dr. Betty Lim, a gifted, compassionate palliative care physician and her colleagues, Des left me and the hundreds if not thousands of lives she had touched over the years. Des's body could no longer battle and she was unable to stave off the final stroke of cancer's end game.

She worked until less than two weeks before she died.

"We must never extend death, Robert," she explained to me not that long before. "We must only extend life." She was talking as the physician, the teacher, and the healer, but in retrospect, she surely was also talking, as well, as the critically ill person she was. She knew she was pushing her body to a point that she would not be able to endure one more procedure.

Des unlocked my potential to love, to live, to be ... and here, in her last moments, she was teaching me what I would need to understand. And yet, after all of our years together – nearly twenty-four - I was never even able to say goodbye. Before slipping into a uremia-induced coma, she looked at me with a bittersweet expression of love, sadness and relief and said, "Robert, I am tired."

"OK, Baby. Rest," I replied. I knew she was asking me to let her go, to take away life support and as much as it hurt me and as much as I wanted to scream "no, not yet...please fight a little longer," I found the courage deep in my heart to give her this last gift from a place of joy for who she was and what she had given me in my life.

I choose not to lessen her pain medication and rouse her so that I could indulge my need to tell her one more time that I loved her or to give her mother, who she also wanted at her bedside, closure. She had also wanted Duncan, our sweet little Yorkie, to be with her and he was, snuggled up against her until the very last moments.

Des had told me so often that when families roused patients who were close to death, it was only for their own benefit, and was never in the best interest of the patient who had finally reached a peaceful place. My Des was in a peaceful place, and I was not about to change that.

She had explained to me that there is a certain type of breathing that occurs before the body is ready to give up and the moment I heard that, I held her in my arms one last time...my glorious, brilliant, courageous wife with whom I shared a love that I thought could only exist in the pages of fiction. Tears rolled down my face and the sighs that came from my body echoed in the room as she stopped breathing. In one last breath, my wonderful wife passed over.

Desiree left an enormous legacy for the medical profession, and she left an enormous legacy for me. She was my teacher, my lover, my friend and my inspiration. She showed me that life is a gift, and we must embrace it with a willing spirit and an open heart. "And above all, we must never forget to be thankful."

I am thankful for all of our years together and thankful that I was given the gift of her love and the time and space to experience it.

Desiree lives in my heart today, as she will for all eternity, for I am beautifully scarred by her love.

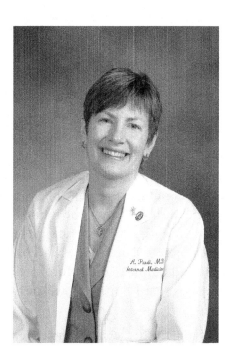

A Message from
Robert Pardi

Thank you for having shared in my wife's journey, a journey of a woman who strove to live life fully regardless of her circumstances and her enormous challenge...a woman who truly chased life.

I was blessed to participate in the evolution of this amazing woman whose entire existence blossomed into an example of learning from life's experiences and embracing the power of choice - the one and only true thing under our control. Desiree's life was an illustration of complete choice - how she wanted to live and how she chose to approach death - demonstrating that a fulfilling life is all about overcoming fear. Together we learned so many lessons about love, life, joy, and purpose, and before leaving you, I wanted to highlight some ideas that I hope you will carry with you going forward.

Desiree viewed Palliative Care as the most rewarding and one of the most essential of all the medical disciplines, defining it as a branch of medicine whose sole purposed it to "optimize quality of life irrespective of a terminal diagnosis." Exactly the way she had lived her own life.

Without question, in 1998, we found ourselves smack dab in the first car of that proverbial emotional rollercoaster. One which set off with an enormous heart-stopping drop leading to a series of corkscrew twists and turns for the next 11-years. And it didn't take long for us to realize that it was our emotions which were molding the *clay of our lives. Yet,* having both learned some tough life lessons as children, allowed us to tap into our resilience and draft a plan of attack: "take no prisoners, move forward with positivity, live consciously and never look back."

As her co-pilot, instinctively and without hesitation, I assumed the roles of caregiver, Rock of Gibraltar, fount of hope, and impromptu Life Coach. It was while learning how to navigate our new terrain that I conceptualized my definition of purpose - *when personal values come into alignment with personal passions.*

Desiree believed she was given the gift of motivation by having to contemplate her death. She fought in the name of her dreams, searched for the daily gifts life offers and, removed what she found unsatisfactory...to have empathy for others and insist on dignity for ourselves. Shouldn't that be how we all live our lives - to find the strength to build and live our lives consciously? To live our lives on purpose and with purpose?

This journey taught me the power of surrendering. I discovered surrendering means letting go of things you cannot control and focusing on things you can. It's all about not attaching our joy to a final outcome but showing up in the here and now. Surrendering, I am convinced, is a true act of bravery. It allows you to be present and express gratitude for each moment. It fuels your resilience and allows you to live authentically.

These and other lessons learned throughout my journey with Des helped me rebuild my own life following her death. Before Desiree was diagnosed, we had made a pact that I would return after she graduated to do "something more meaningful." My pursuit of finance had been motivated by a strong desire to escape a very dysfunctional relationship with my father. Yet, over time, that motivation lost its power. Nonetheless, despite our pact, after her diagnosis I believed it would have been irrational to change careers.

In 2010, a year after Desiree passed away, I returned to my investment banking life in Dubai but as hard as I tried, I could not find my rhythm. My worldview had completely changed. Slowly two latent dreams started to re-emerge: to "do something more meaningful" and to chance living in Italy, which I had been drawn to since childhood. I had watched my wife live her life fully and achieve her dreams. In fact, I dare say Desiree did not live a short life, but rather lived a full 41 years - an accelerated life, in reality.

Having evolved with Des, I believe our life experiences only have value if we share them. So I decided to leave Dubai in 2014 and live life forward. I moved to Italy without a job or a place to live. I didn't know anyone nor speak the language. At the same time, I returned to school to pursue something more purposeful and became a certified Life Coach. I now live in the same small town my great grandfather immigrated from more than 100 years ago and am a practicing Life Coach. I am also a devoted proponent of palliative care, the power of choice and a patient's right to make end-of-life decisions. And I am spreading that message in all facets of my life.

I must thank my wife, Desiree, for her unconditional love and complete sharing of herself with me ... for waking me up to the beauty in life, the joy in ordinary moments and teaching me that the greatest purpose we can ever aspire to is to rise above our own ego and attempt to give everything "we are" to the person we love.

I hope, having walked with me through this journey, you found some nuggets along the way that will motivate you to *Chase Life*. Please remember to embrace life, fully and consciously. It is not about how long you live, but how joyfully you live. This moment shall never come again!

In Memory of Desiree Pardi - I will always love you!

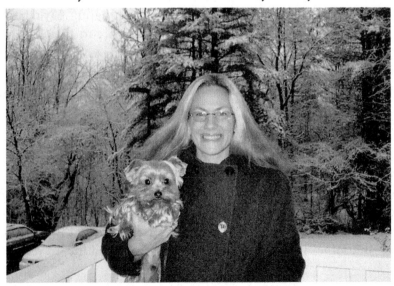

A Message from

Phyllis Melhado

The first time I saw Desiree and Robert Pardi, I knew there was something very special about them. We were at a meditation session being conducted by integrative oncologist Dr. Mitchell Gaynor. I really just wanted to close my eyes and go with the vibration of the Tibetan bowls Dr. Gaynor was playing, but my attention was diverted: I just couldn't stop looking at the attractive young couple seated on the floor several feet away from me. The way the young man held the beautiful young woman in his arms, and the peaceful look she had on her face, said so much.

When we saw each other again at the doctor's office, we struck up a friendship and as I got to know Desiree and Rob, my love and admiration for them both grew. Des's accomplishments as a pioneering palliative care physician were remarkable, and Rob's career in international finance was on a no-holds-barred trajectory. This was a couple that certainly appeared to have it all - with the exception that Desiree was suffering from advanced breast cancer. Had I met them in any other way, I would not have known. Her illness was never discussed. Des put cancer in its place, to be dealt with strictly on a as-needed basis. She did not let it rule her life and it certainly didn't stop her from doing anything. On the contrary, she viewed it as a gift that enabled her to relish the joy possible in life and to give back in a way few of us could ever hope to. She was remarkable.

My friendship with Des and Rob grew and deepened and I learned so much from them about joy and loving and the precious gift of life. When the time came to share their story with the world, I was honored to help Rob do it. His commitment to Des was unlike any I had ever seen, heard of or even read about. Theirs was a love story unlike any other and in that love and the remarkable journey they shared, I know readers will find a source of strength and inspiration, just the way I did.

Acknowledgements

None of this journey would be possible alone. This book would not have been possible without the contribution of many friends, family and colleagues who shared memories, insights and offered enormous encouragement, and for that, we are profoundly grateful. Your support has made all the difference.

Disclaimers

Chasing Life is based on the memories of Robert Pardi. The memories of others may differ.

Conversations have been recreated and certain names, dates, locations and other identifying information have been changed to protect privacy.

About The Authors

Robert Pardi has an MBA in finance from Columbia University and has held various positions in the international arena, including the Abu Dhabi Investment Authority, Dubai-based Evolvence Capitol, and the Swiss School of Management. Well-known in the palliative care community, he is a compelling speaker and has addressed key groups of physicians, nurses, palliative care specialists, hospital administrators and medical students at Columbia Presbyterian Weill Cornell, Memorial 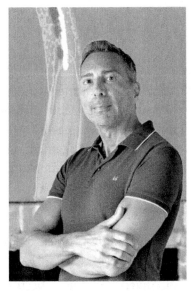 Sloan Kettering and Stony Brook University. After losing his wife to breast cancer, Mr. Pardi re-assessed his life and decided to share the many lessons he learned by becoming a Certified Life Coach. He splits his time between his native New York and Pacentro, Italy. Read more about Robert's work at www.robertpardi.com.

Phyllis Melhado holds a master's degree in Communications from New York University. The author of *The Spa At Lavender Lane*, a 2020 American Fiction Awards Finalist, she has been published in Town & Country, Cosmopolitan and The Scarlet Leaf Literary Review. She has read her work at the legendary NYC Red Room Literary Salon and was the ghost writer of a best-selling health and beauty book as well as a nationally syndicated column. Ms. Melhado is the former Vice President of Pub-

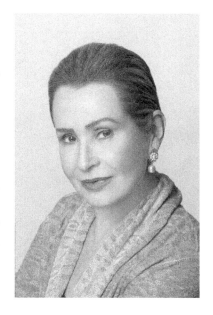

lic Relations for the Estee Lauder Companies. Read more about Phyllis's work at www.phyllismelhado.com.

Made in the USA
Middletown, DE
09 July 2021